"Tired all the Time"

Marie Thomas

"Tired all the Time"

Persistent Fatigue and Healthcare

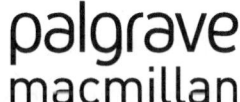

Marie Thomas
Bath Spa University
Bath, UK

ISBN 978-3-319-93912-4   ISBN 978-3-319-93913-1   (eBook)
https://doi.org/10.1007/978-3-319-93913-1

Library of Congress Control Number: 2018947742

Cover illustration: Pattern adapted from an Indian cotton print produced in the 19th
century

This Palgrave Pivot imprint is published by the registered company Springer Nature
Switzerland AG
The registered company address is: Gewerbestrasse 11, 6330 Cham, Switzerland

I continue to be a passionate advocate for research into fatigue not just for CFS but across a range of chronic conditions and dedicate this Pivot to all those who experience persistent fatigue.

PREFACE

The research discussed in this Pivot will centre primarily on two wide-ranging projects: (1) a longitudinal study funded by the Linbury Trust and (2) an evaluation of healthcare provision funded by the Gatsby Foundation. A grant from Healthy Minds at Work funded the three-year follow-up study. The research considered here was conducted as part of the multidisciplinary Cardiff Chronic Fatigue Syndrome (CFS) Project that had a weekly 'CFS Investigation Clinic' supervised by the Section of Infectious Diseases Department of Medicine at the University Hospital of Wales. Patients referred from primary care received a full clinical service at the clinic that assessed features of the disease including the nature and duration of fatigue together with precipitating factors of disease exacerbation. Standard clinical and biochemical investigations were performed in order to exclude other physical diseases presenting as clinical fatigue. Following clinical assessment, patients were invited to join the project's research panel that was supervised by a Health Psychology Research Group. The aim of our research was not to investigate the aetiology of CFS, rather to delineate subgroups within the condition and to examine whether specific outcome measures act as good objective markers of clinical improvement and, more importantly, to explore therapeutic options available to patients.

Chapter 1 charts the medical history of fatigue from neurasthenia in the 1800s to chronic fatigue syndrome (CFS) and discusses three pivotal reports that shaped the nature and direction of research and made recommendations for healthcare provision. Chapter 2 describes the symptoms associated with CFS and the development of a range of subjective and objective measures that can accurately quantify them. Chapter 3 focuses on healthcare provision for people with CFS including a survey of patient and GP beliefs together with possible pharmacological and behavioural therapies to manage symptoms of the illness. Chapter 4 considers fatigue as a secondary but significant symptom in chronic conditions and describes the fatigue reported by adults with the neurodevelopmental disorder, developmental coordination disorder (DCD). Chapter 5 offers an overview of the research described in Chaps. 2, 3 and 4 and makes recommendations for future research.

Bath Spa University, UK   Marie Thomas

ACKNOWLEDGEMENTS

To Andy Smith, whose mentorship, guidance and encouragement continues to drive me forward. To Dr Llewelyn and Mr Sadlier for affording me the opportunity to attend consultations and for imparting their substantial knowledge and insight into the illness that is CFS. To my husband, whose love and support sustains me. Most importantly, to all the people who took part in my research and continue to do so.

CONTENTS

List of Abbreviations

AfME	Action for ME
CBT	Cognitive Behaviour Therapy
CDC	Centers for Disease Control and Prevention
CFIDS	Chronic Fatigue and Immune Deficiency Syndrome
CFQ	Cognitive Failures Questionnaire
CFS	Chronic Fatigue Syndrome
CMO	Chief Medical Officer
CNS	Central Nervous System
CSH	Current State of Health
DCD	Developmental Coordination Disorder
EBV	Epstein–Barr Virus
ECG	Electrocardiogram
EMG	Electromyography
FM	Fibromyalgia
GET	Graded Exercise Therapy
GP	General Practitioner
MAOI	Monoamine-oxidase Inhibitor
MCT	Multi Convergent Therapy
ME	Myalgic Encephalomyelitis
MRI	Magnetic Resonance Imaging
MS	Multiple Sclerosis
Msec	Milli-seconds
NHS	National Health Service
NICE	National Institute for health and Care Excellence
NMR	Nuclear Magnetic Resonance
OT	Occupational Therapy
PD	Parkinson's Disease

PFRS	Profile of Fatigue-Related Symptoms
PIFS	Post-infectious Fatigue Syndrome
PVFS	Post-viral Fatigue Syndrome
RA	Rheumatoid Arthritis
RCT	Randomised Controlled Trial
SNRI	Serotonin/Noradrenalin Re-uptake Inhibitors
SSRI	Selective Serotonin Re-uptake Inhibitors
TD	Typically Developing
URTI	Upper Respiratory Tract Infection

LIST OF TABLES

CHAPTER 1

A Medical History of Chronic Fatigue

Abstract This chapter provides an insight into the depth of the problem that fatigue poses to society by chronicling its medical history from neurasthenia in the 1800s to Chronic Fatigue Syndrome (CFS). The chapter also discusses three pivotal reports about chronic fatigue which were published in the 1990s. The first of these reports went on to shape the nature and direction of research in the UK. The second report suggested the nomenclature of the illness and called for physicians to acknowledge the condition and offer a patient service. The third report continued to make recommendation for healthcare provision by suggesting possible intervention for CFS.

Keywords Neurasthenia • Post-viral fatigue syndrome • Myalgic encephalomyelitis • Chronic fatigue syndrome • Guidelines for research

Fatigue is the normal result of over-exertion or lack of sleep and is defined as 'extreme tiredness resulting from mental or physical exertion or illness' (*Oxford English Dictionary*, 2017). Individuals experience an intense subjective sense of tiredness, energy depletion and weakness. Whether it is physical and/or cognitive in nature, fatigue can be interpreted differently by different individuals, ranging from tiredness to clinically relevant exhaustion. This makes the symptom difficult to quantify. It is also subjective. That is to say, the interpretation of the fatigue experienced is based

© The Author(s) 2018
M. Thomas, *"Tired all the Time"*,
https://doi.org/10.1007/978-3-319-93913-1_1

on an individual's personal opinion, interpretation, point of view, emotion and judgement. However, when it persists over time (i.e. is chronic in nature) and is unresolved by rest, fatigue can be extremely debilitating.

In order to understand the increasing problem chronic fatigue presents to healthcare, it is important first to consider the historical context. Although often thought of as an illness that emerged in the 1980s, chronic fatigue has been redefined over time, and this is reflected in the changes in nomenclature used to describe it and the way in which the scientific community has chosen to research it. In the early 1990s, Wessely presented an historical background of post-viral fatigue syndrome (PVFS) in the *British Medical Bulletin* (Wessely, 1991). This in-depth essay charted the appearance of the illness in the medical literature and went some way to explain the cultural attitudes towards chronic fatigue in society. An overview of the salient points will be presented here to put its importance in the medical and research literature into perspective (Thomas, 2009).

The history of chronic fatigue stretches back over one hundred years. Its appearance in the medical literature as *neurasthenia* can be traced back to the mid-nineteenth century. Described as a weakness in the nervous system, a diagnosis of neurasthenia was grounded in neurology, an emerging discipline. Seen almost as a badge of honour by experts and those diagnosed the condition at that time, neurasthenia was associated with hard-working, intellectual men from the higher social classes. Its increasing prevalence was ascribed to the ascent of capitalism and the raised expectations it produced and emphasis on personal productivity.

By the beginning of the twentieth century, it was viewed as exhaustion of the central nervous system (CNS) and attributed to a range of aetiologies including deficient energy sources, a genetic fault or as the result of toxic, metabolic or infective insults (Cobb, 1920; Forster, 1900; Pershing, 1904). As a consequence, clinicians postulated that treatments aiming to stimulate the CNS or sedate over-activity and/or those which might replace or recuperate lost energy would address symptoms. The suggested methods for replacing or recuperating energy included the application of electrical stimuli and the rest cure.

Dissenters then began to challenge the existence of an organic cause of neurasthenia, and the search for an aetiological explanation moved towards the then emerging discipline of psychiatry. Modifications to the definition of the illness also shifted to include mild melancholic, anxious or depressive states and proffered existing treatments with appropriate modifications.

The absence of a known cellular basis for the fatigue also led to clinicians asserting that the rest cure was ill-advised and unnecessary. Instead, activity or exercise along with psychotherapy were being suggested (Hall, 1905). A shift in terminology also occurred. Physical nomenclature such as 'painful fatigue' were being replaced with psychological terms such as 'anhedonia' (Myerson, 1922). By 1941, neurasthenia was described as being 'in reality depression—perhaps minor, attenuated, atypical, masked, but always forms of anxious melancholia' (Tinel, 1941, p. 926).

Notwithstanding, researchers continued to search for the thus far elusive organic cause of this chronic fatigue. Following on from suggestions by Van Deusen (1869), for example, that neurasthenia was a toxic state linked to an infective agent, the focus returned to the possible involvement of specific infectious agents such as influenza in triggering chronic fatigue. This association led to the emergence of the term post-viral fatigue syndrome (PVFS). However, it was later made clear that this fatigue state could follow any viral infection where anxiety and/or depression were a comorbid condition (Ash, 1909; Lane, 1906).

Despite this setback, researchers continued to pursue an aetiology based on infection until as recently as the 1980s. Straus and colleagues reported findings that suggested the causative agent of chronic fatigue was the Epstein–Barr virus (EBV) which causes infectious mononucleosis—also referred to as glandular fever (Straus et al., 1985). This association between a specific virus and fatigue led to the introduction of the label chronic Epstein–Barr infection. However, although glandular fever is very often accompanied by prolonged fatigue, this usually resolves within a six-month period post-infection.

Probably one of the most well-known terms associated with chronic fatigue in the medical history of the condition has been myalgic encephalomyelitis (ME). This diagnosis is also the one which has generated great interest within the scientific community and society. The first reported case of ME appeared in 1955 following a mysterious outbreak of a fatiguing illness which afflicted the majority of staff at the Royal Free Hospital in London—which was later documented by Ramsay in 1986 (Ramsay, 1986). This benign condition—encephalomyelitis—was thought to have its origins within the discipline of infectious diseases (Medical Staff of the Royal Free Hospital, 1976). The claims of the infectious nature of ME proved difficult to substantiate and, whilst agreeing that the outbreak was contagious, was famously contradicted by McEvedy and Beard (1970) who considered that the contagion was one of mass hysteria. The aetiology of ME remains contentious as neither view point has been corroborated and the matter remains unresolved. Although this could be disconcerting for those who experience such chronic fatigue, in the grand tradition of science, it did provide impetus for ongoing research that would ultimately lead to a better understanding of the origins of and mechanism behind this insidious condition.

Although sporadic cases of ME continued, its incidence as an epidemic waned over time (Smith, 1989). Intermittent cases of the condition became more widespread in the 1980s and the outlook for individuals with this condition became bleak. Again, appearing to mimic the history of neurasthenia, the fatigue experienced in ME was at first thought to be neuromuscular in origin and treatments once again centred on the rest cure. However, although the theories put forward were supported by data from electromyography (EMG) and nuclear magnetic resonance (NMR) studies, as reported in a review by Jamal and Millar (1991), there was some doubt as to their validity. Research then focussed on a possible aetiology involving changes in the CNS. When this direction of enquiry proved fruitless, and, in almost a repeat of what occurred previously in the history of unexplained fatigue, the aetiological route of ME finally arrived at the psychological direction.

The term Chronic Fatigue Syndrome (CFS) first appeared in the medical literature in 1988 in both the USA and Australia (Holmes et al., 1988; Lloyd, Wakefield, Boughton, & Dwyer, 1988; Straus et al., 1988). In the USA, it was also referred to as chronic fatigue and immune deficiency syndrome (CFIDS) by patient groups. In a departure from the history of neurasthenia and ME, the initial focus of research into the aetiology of CFS returned to focus on the role of viruses, namely the EBV—as investigated previously in the USA (Straus et al., 1985)—and enteroviruses—originally the polio virus—in the UK.

Again, however, this substantial body of research conducted over several years, aiming to identify not only a causative agent but biological diagnostic markers, was to no avail. Early reports of an association between chronic fatigue and a number of possible causative infective agents generated hope that an aetiology was imminent, and a treatment would closely follow. Unfortunately, these claims have yet to be substantiated (Dismukes, Wade, Lee, Dockery, & Hain, 1990; Straus et al., 1988). Nevertheless, it was thought that persistent viral infection could be a possible mechanism for perpetuation of the illness (Archard, Bowles, Behan, Bell, & Doyle, 1988; Bowles, 1993; Cunningham, Bowles, Lane, Dubowitz, & Archard, 1990).

This was corroborated in some part by studies indicating increased susceptibility to infections in patients suffering psychological stress which might also explain the circumstances seen in CFS (Cohen, Tyrrell, Russell, Jarvis, & Smith, 1993; Cohen, Tyrrell, & Smith, 1991; Cohen & Williamson, 1991). In fact, a major impact of the disease on the patient has been described as one of a 'chronic, recurring, flu-like illness' (Dubois et al., 1984; Jones et al., 1985; Komaroff, 1991; Straus et al., 1988). Anecdotally, patients with CFS were frequently reporting symptoms which seemed to indicate recurrent infections and it was postulated that these infections could be implicated as a possible means whereby the illness is exacerbated (Smith, 1991). These claims were not tested under controlled experimental conditions until much later on and will be expanded upon in Chap. 2.

The continued lack of evidence indicating an organic basis for CFS did not result in a decline in scientific interest. With the increase in the incidence of CFS in the UK, primary and secondary healthcare providers were being put under increasing pressure to offer a service to patients with this condition. In order for the NHS to provide this service, it was necessary that research was carried out to both understand the factors associated with the illness and also identify factors responsible for perpetuating. In addition, there was a need to develop an appropriate strategy for managing the condition. Three pivotal publications were influential in shaping the direction of research and the development of management strategies in the UK. These were (1) the Guidelines for Research (Sharpe et al., 1991), (2) the Joint Working Committee of Royal Colleges of Physicians, Psychiatrists and General Practitioners (1996) and (3) the CFS/ME Working Group (2002) reports.

The Guidelines for Research were produced following a meeting of leading CFS experts in Oxford in 1990 (Sharpe et al., 1991). The aim of the meeting was to facilitate consensus between different UK research groups for both conducting research and disseminating the findings. The resulting document also provided a series of proposals to bring clarity to the contradictory findings from previous multidisciplinary studies, in order to agree on which patients should be included in the research and on the minimal data that should be reported. It was acknowledged that research into CFS was increasingly being conducted by clinicians and academics from an increasingly diverse range of disciplines, thus making comparisons between studies largely impossible. The members of the group recognised that, 'Agreement on case definition and assessment methods is necessary if progress is to be made' (Sharpe et al., 1991, p. 118).

The need to develop a case definition was important as there had been a range of illnesses included within the syndrome including benign ME, chronic infectious mononucleosis, PVFS, the infection at the Royal Free Hospital and CFS. This led to a lack of consensus when describing the groups of patients being studied as these conditions present with similar symptom patterns but differ sufficiently to make meaningful comparison between studies unsuccessful. Other barriers to tangible agreement in the research include how the patients were recruited and from where, how the studies were designed, who the patients group was being compared to and what measures were being used to compare them (Sharpe et al., 1991).

In order to bring coherence to future research, the report set out a preliminary glossary of terms defining five main symptoms experienced by patients: (1) fatigue, (2) disability, (3) mood disturbance, (4) muscle pain (myalgia) and (5) sleep disturbance. It was also recommended that these five symptoms should be considered and described separately. For example, the fatigue experienced in CFS can be both mental—such as low alertness—and physical—such as a lack of energy or strength in the muscles. It would also be important to define how each symptom is distinguished from others—for example, the distinction between fatigue and low mood. Next, criteria for rating each symptom's presence were set out—such as the effects of a symptom on a person's daily functioning. Finally, it was necessary to attempt to describe each symptom in additional detail—for example, fatigue could be described as mild, moderate or severe.

Although it was acknowledged that there were no clinical signs that could be used to characterise the illness, it was suggested that the absence or presence of signs should be documented. In terms of how the illness should be referred to (i.e. its nomenclature), two syndromes were proposed: (1) CFS or (2) post-infectious fatigue syndrome (PIFS). PIFS was suggested as the preferred term for a subtype of CFS which followed or was associated with a definite infective episode. A major historic milestone in our understanding of CFS that arose from this meeting was the proposed and agreed diagnostic benchmark which formed the basis of the Oxford criteria (Sharpe et al., 1991).

As indicated above, other salient issues which acted as barriers to conceptual conformity in CFS research was sampling (recruitment) bias. The guidelines recommended two methods of patient recruitment—proposed randomisation and consecutive referral. Two study designs were also suggested: (1) cross-sectional in order to establish associations within the illness and (2) longitudinal to look at how the illness progressed over time.

Finally, the report stressed the need to develop reliable, valid and reproducible measures to assess the illness, such as subjective measures of fatigue and disability.

The 1990 meeting was attended by the two research leads of what later became the Cardiff CFS Project and were co-authors of the consensus report. In Chap. 2, the way in which we addressed some of the report's recommendations in the years that followed will be discussed.

Although the guidelines for research acknowledged the existence of the illness, the absence of a possible cause and diagnostic tool meant that certain sections of the medical profession were unwilling to view CFS as a genuine illness. General practitioners (GPs) are the gatekeepers to accessing secondary healthcare services. Practitioners sceptical about the validity of a CFS diagnosis might be less likely to refer patients to secondary care. Indeed, anecdotal accounts from patients taking part in our research confirmed that this was happening quite frequently. To further investigate these accounts, a study was conducted to explore the illness beliefs of patients and GPs and this is discussed in Chap. 3.

To address patient concerns, the English chief medical officer (CMO) established a Joint Working Group Committee made up of members of the Royal Colleges of Physicians, Psychiatrists and General Practitioners who had experience of CFS both in clinical practice and research (Royal Colleges of Physicians, Psychiatrists and General Practitioners, 1996; Wessely, 1996). The committee was set up to develop recommendations grounded in evidence-based medicine and so supported by published data.

The general consensus of the joint Working Group was that CFS was the most appropriate term for the illness. Their reasons for this being that, 'This can be operationally defined, a prerequisite for clinical research. It is a short and accurate label, free from unproven aetiological claims' (Wessely, 1996, p. 498). The committee chose this label over ME as it was believed that ME 'erroneously endorses the existence of a specific pathology for which there is no evidence' (Wessely, 1996, p. 498). The joint Working Group reiterated that there was a lack of scientific evidence to link the role of viral infections in causing CFS and agreed that the illness had both a physical and mental aetiology. A caveat being that an infection by the EBV may result in chronic fatigue. The report also recommended that the existence and nature of the cognitive impairments associated with the illness should be fully investigated. In terms of service provision, the committee endorsed a multidisciplinary approach to management programmes in order to address the needs of the individual patient. Healthcare providers were urged to keep up to date with the emerging evidence to ensure the promotion of good doctor-patient relationships and recommended that the majority of cases should be managed in primary care.

The report was not well received by some mainly due to the recommendation that the term CFS should replace ME, as it was believed that this implied an overemphasis on the psychological aspects of the illness. Taking the concerns by patients, carers and voluntary organisations into account, the CMO commissioned a new Working Group in 1998. The CFS/ME Working Group widened participation to include not only physicians, but also patients, carers and support groups.

The brief of the CFS/ME Working Group was to conduct a comprehensive review of practice and management in order to develop best practice guidance for the treatment and care of patients. Their report was aimed at professionals, patients and carers alike (CFS/ME Working Group, 2002). The Working Group identified five areas of concern that needed to be addressed: (1) recognition that ME/CFS exists, with a review of the terminology used by clinicians; (2) improvements in the knowledge base of healthcare professionals around the management of the illness and the support of patients; (3) increasing the level of specialist expertise available; (4) provision of secondary and tertiary care service with appropriate training and education for healthcare professionals; (5) a need for further cross-disciplinary research.

When considering the direction of research, the Working Group identified several areas of interest. These included the aetiology, pathogenesis, epidemiology and natural history of the illness together with the identification of subgroups, the efficacy of interventions and symptom management and the development of outcome measures for use in both clinical and research settings. The report, once again, acknowledged that there was no cure for CFS. They did, however, identify cognitive behaviour therapy (CBT), graded exercise and pacing (where the individual strikes a balance between activity and rest in order to conserve energy) as possible management strategies. Comparisons between the benefits of counselling and these three rehabilitative approaches were also recommended (CFS/ME Working Group, 2002). Clinicians were also advised to refer to evidence-based practice when managing their patients. The efficacy of CBT, graded exercise therapy (GET) and counselling for alleviating the symptoms associated with CFS will be discussed in Chap. 3.

The Working Group report courted controversy as it appeared to suggest that scientific knowledge around CFS had not advanced a great deal since the Oxford consensus meeting guidelines (Sharpe et al., 1991) and that that illness management and the way in which healthcare professionals viewed CFS had not altered despite the recommendations in the 1996 report (Royal Colleges of Physicians, Psychiatrists and General Practitioners, 1996). Publication of the Working Group report was delayed following the resignation of four key group members—two psychiatrists, a public health doctor and a nurse therapist. The reasons given for their decision included (1) the focus of the report being the medical model and the downplaying of the psychological and social factors associated with the condition and (2) the inclusion of pacing as a management strategy which had not been assessed under trial conditions (Eaton, 2002a). Two patient representatives also resigned while the report was being compiled due to the recommendation that CBT and graded exercise should be used in the management of CFS (Eaton, 2002b). Further concerns were raised about the use of the 'compromise' term CFS/ME following the publication of the report (Sharpe, 2002) and there were some worries that the report's conclusions were based on anecdotal rather than scientific evidence (Straus, 2002). Despite the controversy surrounding the 2002 Working Group report, the Government announced an £8.5 million fund to develop clinical services for patients with CFS in the UK.

SUMMARY

Throughout its history, chronic fatigue in its different forms has confounded the medical profession, researchers, patients, carers and health service policy makers alike. The fatigue experienced is excessive and is not resolved by rest or sleep. There is no clear aetiology, no clinical diagnostic tool and no cure.

The meeting of experts in Oxford attributed the lack of consensus between research studies in the UK to several methodological flaws. The group developed a set of guidelines which aimed to facilitate comparability between studies and to recommend ways in which research could develop, such as the need to identify and investigate factors responsible for both causing and perpetuating the illness. The guidelines purposefully did not aim to enter the 'organic versus psychological cause' debate, rather it set out to develop a working case definition, thereby providing a gold standard for researchers when recruiting CFS patients to their studies (Sharpe et al., 1991).

The Royal Colleges report agreed the use of the term chronic fatigue syndrome which was not popular amongst patients, carers and support groups. They did, however, urge clinicians to accept the existence of the illness, provide a service for patients and take steps to manage patients in their care. The report concluded that CFS would be better managed by multidisciplinary healthcare teams (Royal Colleges of Physicians, Psychiatrists and General Practitioners, 1996).

In the absence of a cure, the CFS/ME Working Group recommended that CBT and graded exercise were the most successful methods for managing symptoms of the illness and repeated the Royal Colleges' call for the development of multidisciplinary teams of healthcare professionals offering individualised treatment programmes designed to best suit the patients' needs (CFS/ME Working Group, 2002).

The following chapters (Chaps. 2 and 3) will describe and discuss how we addressed the recommendations of these three pivotal reports namely, the investigation of the wide range of symptoms associated with CFS and recovery in the untreated illness, the development of outcome measures and their subsequent use in the evaluation of the efficacy of interventions to manage the illness.

REFERENCES

Archard, D. V., Bowles, N. E., Behan, P. O., Bell, E. J., & Doyle, D. (1988). Postviral fatigue syndrome: Persistence of enterovirus RNA in muscle and elevated creatine kinase. *Journal of Social Medicine, 81*, 326–329.

Ash, E. (1909). Nervous breakdown: The disease of our age. *Medical Times, 37*, 35–54.

Bowles, N. E. (1993). Persistence of enterovirus RNA in muscle biopsy samples suggests that some cases of chronic fatigue syndrome result from a previous inflammatory viral myopathy. *Journal of Medicine, 24*, 59–65.

CFS/ME Working Group. (2002). *Report to the Chief Medical Officer of an independent working group*. London: Department of Health.

Cobb, I. (1920). *A manual of neurasthenia (nervous exhaustion)*. London: Bailliere, Tindall and Cox.

Cohen, S., Tyrrell, D. A., Russell, M. A. H., Jarvis, M. J., & Smith, A. P. (1993). Smoking, alcohol consumption and susceptibility to the common cold. *American Journal of Public Health, 83*, 1277–1281.

Cohen, S., Tyrrell, D. A., & Smith, A. P. (1991). Psychological stress and susceptibility to the common cold. *New England Journal of Medicine, 325*, 606–612.

Cohen, S., & Williamson, G. (1991). Stress and infectious disease in humans. *Psychological Bulletin, 109*, 5–24.

Cunningham, L., Bowles, N. E., Lane, R. J. H., Dubowitz, V., & Archard, L. C. (1990). Persistence of enterovirus RNA in chronic fatigue syndrome is associated with the abnormal production of equal amounts of positive and negative strands of enteroviral RNA. *Journal of General Virology, 71*, 1399–1402.

Dismukes, W. E., Wade, J. S., Lee, J. Y., Dockery, B. K., & Hain, J. D. (1990). A randomised, double-blind trial of nystatin therapy for the candidiasis hypersensitivity syndrome. *New England Journal of Medicine, 323*, 1717–1723.

Dubois, R., Seeley, J., Brus, I., Sakamoto, K., Ballow, M., Harada, S., et al. (1984). Chronic mononucleosis syndrome. *Southern Medical Journal, 77*, 1376–1382.

Eaton, L. (2002a). Chronic fatigue report delayed as row breaks out over content. *British Medical Journal, 324*, 7.

Eaton, L. (2002b). Recognising chronic fatigue is key to improving outcomes. *British Medical Journal, 324*, 131.

Forster, G. (1900). Common features in Neurasthenia and insanity: Their common basis and common treatment. *American Journal of Insanity, 56*, 395–418.

Hall, H. (1905). The systematic use of work as a remedy in Neurasthenia and allied conditions. *Boston Medical Surgery Journal, 152*, 29–31.

Holmes, G. P., Kaplan, J. E., Gantz, N. M., Komaroff, A. L., Schonberger, L. B., Straus, S. E., et al. (1988). CFS: A working case definition. *Annals Internal Medicine, 108*, 387–389.

Jamal, G. A., & Millar, R. G. (1991). Neurophysiology of postviral fatigue syndrome. *British Medical Bulletin, 47*, 815–825.

Jones, J. F., Ray, C. G., Minnich, L. L., Hicks, M. J., Kibler, R., & Lucas, D. O. (1985). Evidence of active Epstein-Barr virus infection in patients with persistent, unexplained illnesses: Elevated anti-early antigen antibodies. *Annals of Internal Medicine, 102*, 1–7.

Komaroff, A. L. (1991). Postviral fatigue syndrome: A review of American research and practice. In R. Jenkins & J. Mowbray (Eds.), *Post-viral fatigue syndrome (ME)* (pp. 41–59). Chichester: Wiley.

Lane, C. (1906). The mental element in the etiology of neurasthenia. *Journal of Nervous Mental Disorders, 33*, 463–466.

Lloyd, A., Wakefield, D., Boughton, C., & Dwyer, J. (1988). What is myaligic encephalomyelitis. *Lancet, 1*, 1286–1287.

McEvedy, C., & Beard, A. (1970). Royal free epidemic of 1955: A reconsideration. *British Medical Journal, 1*, 7–11.

Medical Staff of the Royal Free Hospital. (1976). An outbreak of encephalomyelitis in the Royal Free Hospital Group, London, in 1955. *British Medical Journal, 2*, 895–904.

Myerson, A. (1922). Adhedonia. *American Journal of Psychiatry, 2,* 87–103.

Oxford English Dictionary. (2017). Oxford: Oxford University Press.

Pershing, H. (1904). The treatment of Neurasthenia. *Medical News, 84,* 637–640.

Ramsay, M. (1986). *Postviral fatigue syndrome: The saga of Royal Free Disease.* London: Gower Medical.

Report of the Royal Colleges of Physicians, Psychiatrists and General Practitioners. (1996). *Chronic Fatigue Syndrome.* London: RCP.

Sharpe, M. (2002). The English chief medical officer's working parties' report on the management of CFS/ME: Significant breakthrough or unsatisfactory compromise. *Journal of Psychosomatic Research, 52,* 437–438.

Sharpe, M. C., Archard, L. C., Banatvala, J. E., Borysiewicz, L. K., Clare, A. W., David, A., et al. (1991). A report—Chronic fatigue syndrome: Guidelines for research. *Journal of the Royal Society of Medicine, 84,* 118–121.

Smith, A. P. (1991). Cognitive changes in ME. In R. Jenkins & J. Mowbray (Eds.), *Post-viral fatigue syndrome (ME)* (pp. 179–194). Chichester: Wiley.

Smith, D. (1989). *Understanding M.E.* London: Robinson Publishing.

Straus, S. E. (2002). Caring for patients with Chronic Fatigue Syndrome. *British Medical Journal, 324,* 124–125.

Straus, S. E., Dale, J. K., Tobi, M., Lawley, T., Preble, O., Blaese, R. M., et al. (1988). Acyclovir treatment of the CFS: Lack of efficacy in a placebo-controlled trial. *New England Journal of Medicine, 319,* 1692–1698.

Straus, S., Tosato, G., Armstrong, G., Lawley, T., Preble, O. T., Henle, W., et al. (1985). Persisting illness and fatigue in adults with evidence of Epstein-Barr virus infection. *Annals of Internal Medicine, 102,* 7–16.

Thomas, M. (2009). *Exploring the beliefs and underlying functional deficits associated with CFS and the identification of predictors of recovery and successful illness management.* PhD thesis, University of Wales.

Tinel, J. (1941). *Conceptions et traitement des états neurasthéniques.* Paris: JB Bailliére et Fils.

Van Deusen, E. (1869). Observation on a form of nervous prostration (Neurasthenia) culminating in insanity. *American Journal of Insanity, 25,* 445–461.

Wessely, S. (1991). History of postviral fatigue syndrome. *British Medical Bulletin, 47,* 919–941.

Wessely, S. (1996). CFS: Summary of a report of a joint committee of the Royal Colleges of Physicians, Psychiatrists and General Practitioners. *Journal of the Royal Colleges of Physicians of London, 30,* 497–504.

CHAPTER 2

Chronic Fatigue Syndrome

Abstract This chapter discusses the diagnostic criteria for CFS, its prevalence and recovery in the untreated condition. The chapter goes on to
describe research conducted to investigate the impairments associated
with the condition in line with the 1991 Guidelines for Research. A
range of individual symptoms associated with both physical and mental
fatigue is discussed together with illness severity and comorbid symptoms. The chapter concludes with the results of a comparison study
including a major breakthrough in the identification of objective cognitive impairments in CFS.

Keywords Chronic fatigue syndrome • Fatigue • Cognition • Sleep •
Mood • Psychosocial factors

The fatigue experienced in chronic fatigue syndrome (CFS) is not only of
sufficient severity to cause substantial functional impairment, it is also
accompanied by four or more coexisting symptoms including those of a
cognitive or neuropsychiatric nature (Fukuda et al., 1994). The illness by
definition must be of at least six months duration with the potential for it to
become debilitating and persistent (Andersen, Permin, & Albrecht, 2004).

Fatiguing illnesses are difficult conditions to accurately assess and diagnose. This is due to fatigue being largely subjective in nature, meaning
different things to different people. The term itself describes conditions

© The Author(s) 2018
M. Thomas, *"Tired all the Time"*,
https://doi.org/10.1007/978-3-319-93913-1_2

ranging from moderate tiredness to clinical exhaustion. As mentioned in Chap. 1—which focussed on the historical development of fatigue—a working case definition for CFS was developed in 1988 by Holmes and colleagues which provided a structured way of categorising the illness (Holmes et al., 1988).

The following sections will provide an overview of the research which set out to develop working case definitions in both the UK and the USA, as well as to estimate prevalence of the syndrome and investigate prognosis for recovery in the untreated illness. This chapter then will focus on two studies—Thomas and Smith (2006, 2008)—which discuss the symptoms associated with CFS, possible underlying mechanisms that might perpetuate it, recovery in the untreated patient, and the identification of possible CFS subgroups.

The Thomas and Smith (2008) study aimed to address criticisms of previous research. There had also been some concern that relatively low numbers of individuals had been studied and, due to the heterogeneity of the illness, there was poor experimental power. To address this, over 300 patients fitting the CDC criteria (Fukuda et al., 1994) were recruited to the study. Others had criticised the lack of appropriate control groups and we addressed this by recruiting 126 healthy volunteers from a cross section of the general population. This healthy control group was (1) demographically matched to the patient group and (2) they completed a similar screening process. Concerns voiced by Wearden and Appleby (1996) regarding validity of using objective measures of cognitive performance for this patient group were addressed by administering tasks which not only reflected the type of cognitive impairments reported by the patients, but were tests that had been used in previous studies of the illness (Smith, Pollock, Thomas, Llewelyn, & Borysiewicz, 1996; Smith et al., 1999) and in studies of fatigue in healthy individuals (Smith, Brockman, Flynn, Maben, & Thomas, 1993).

DEFINITION

In 1990, a meeting of clinicians and researchers in Oxford led to a modification of the Holmes et al. CFS case definition (Holmes et al., 1988) and came to a consensus regarding the nature and direction of future research (Sharpe et al., 1991). In the USA, the Centre for Disease Control and Prevention (CDC) criteria provided further coherence and guidelines for clinicians and researchers in the field (Fukuda et al., 1994). The resulting criteria define a person with CFS as one who has experienced persistent, debilitating fatigue for six months or more which is not resolved by rest and is not due to ongoing exertion. The onset of fatigue is described here as 'definite' or 'new' and there may be several coexisting physical and mental symptoms present.

There is a substantial decrease in personal, social and occupational activities for individuals with CFS which severely affects their quality of life. In addition, the financial cost in terms of loss of employment and increased uptake of healthcare resources are significant. It was important, therefore, to conduct studies into the causes, aetiology and clinical features of CFS in order to aid diagnosis and develop possible treatment protocols. Reports by patients of impaired cognition were also investigated to discover both the level of impairment in CFS and the possible mechanisms underlying these effects.

PREVALENCE

Early research in to the prevalence of CFS suggests that the incidence of the illness in the general population is relatively low (Afari & Buchwald, 2003; Price, North, Wessely, & Fraser, 1992; Ranjith, 2005). That being said, this relatively low prevalence should in no way detract from the severe effect the illness has on the individual's quality of life. Decreased personal, occupational and social activities combine to instil a sense of frustration and hopelessness within the patient. In addition, financial concerns were raised about the increased uptake of unemployment benefits, increased sickness absence and the increasing cost to healthcare resources caused by the illness. To quantify this, a surveillance study conducted by the CDC estimated that the cost in terms of lost productivity, per year, for each patient with CFS in the USA was $20,000 (Reyes et al., 1999). This relatively high cost acted as an important driver for continued research into the causes of and potential therapies for CFS as a way to reduce the financial burden reported (Reynolds, Vernon, Bouchery, & Reeves, 2004).

PROGNOSIS

Early on in the history of CFS research, studies mainly concentrated on investigations into the long-term prognosis of the condition as there were no coherent treatment protocols in place. Studies that were longitudinal in nature attempted to calculate recovery rates and identify factors associated with CFS that could possibly be used to predict positive outcome or recovery. As with other heterogeneous conditions, early predictions of recovery rates in the untreated illness produced contradictory findings. It was concluded that the variability in recovery rate data were due to the use of differing criteria to define recovery in the patient group. In one study, for example, recovery or remission was described as (1) an individual no longer experiencing fatigue, (2) someone experiencing less than the required four associated CFS symptoms and (3) an individual that no longer reported impairments that interfered with daily activities (Reyes et al., 1999). When applying these conditions, a spontaneous recovery rate of 31.4% was reported during the first five years of the illness. Russo and colleagues followed 98 referrals to a specialised CFS clinic and found that, although a relatively large number of patients (41%) experienced moderate to complete recovery up to three years after their illness began, only 2.6% of these rated themselves as being 'fully recovered'. However, 29.5% of the patient sample felt well enough to return to work during this three-year period (Russo et al., 1998). On reviewing the research literature, Cairns and Hotopf (2005) highlighted the inconsistencies in the reporting of recovery and concluded that, although improvement in patients at follow-up varied considerably, ranging considerably from 8% to 63% depending on the source, full recovery from the illness was actually quite rare. As we will see later in the chapter, our research concurs with reports of the low spontaneous recovery rate in both the short and longer term (Thomas & Smith, 2006; Thomas, 2009).

As touched on above, one of the problems in measuring recovery in CFS is that patients often go through periods of remission throughout the life course of the condition. Remission is often seen in those who have only had the illness for a short period of time (Reyes et al., 1999; Nisenbaum, Jones, Jones, & Reeves, 2000). In order to achieve a clearer picture, it was suggested that several independent illness-related measures of recovery should be used to try to differentiate between remission and true recovery. Another factor to be taken into consideration when reporting recovery data in longitudinal studies is that it cannot be presumed that the patients questioned did not attend some form of intervention during the prevailing time period—such as behavioural or pharmacological interventions. The caveat to this being that formal treatment was not available at that time, so the natural progression of the illness is being discussed.

In a longitudinal study of 307 patients recruited from a specialised outpatient clinic (Thomas & Smith, 2006; Thomas, 2009), we asked patients with CFS to rate their health on a self-report scale. This current state of health (CSH) scale consisted of the following five items: (1) worse than at any time, (2) bad, (3) bad with some recovery, (4) recovering with occasional relapses and (5) almost completely recovered. Patients completed this scale at their initial clinic visit, at their 6-month follow-up clinic visit, 18 months after their initial visit and at three years. When looking at these data, 2% of respondents reported being 'almost completely recovered' at the six-month time point which rose to 6% at three years, thereby providing further evidence of the low recovery rate in the untreated illness.

In terms of factors associated with recovery in the untreated illness, those who were younger at the onset of the illness had fewer physical symptoms associated with the condition, had better mental and general health, low levels of emotional distress, and were more likely to recover (Russo et al., 1998). Not surprisingly, a systematic review by Cairns and Hotopf (2005) found that a relatively low level of fatigue at illness onset was linked with more favourable outcomes. Of additional interest was the finding that a sense of control over the symptoms associated with the illness and the acknowledgement that the cause of the illness may not be physical significantly improved prognosis (Cairns & Hotopf, 2005). Furthermore, several aspects of the disorder such as psychopathology, ratings of well-being, psychosocial and demographic factors have been implicated in the outcome (Smith et al., 1996). Previous studies have also indicated that there were possible confounding variables which affected the severity of CFS including psychosocial factors, support mechanisms, health measures, psychopathology and cognition (Smith et al., 1996, 1999). These findings emphasised the importance of considering this condition from within a biopsychosocial framework. The biopsychosocial model was first introduced by Engel (1980) and explains how biological, psychological, interpersonal and individual circumstances affect health over time. Examples of biological factors include immunological, cardiac and neurological systems which are vital to the health of the whole body. The psychological factors in the model include cognitive, emotional, motivational, attitudinal and behavioural systems that can affect health. Examples of interpersonal factors include the way in which actual or perceived social interactions affect health. This could be influenced by the communication style of a clinician or peer pressure. Circumstantial or contextual factors include shared culture, norms and values together with healthcare policies.

The aspects of CFS described above are discussed in more detail in the following section which relates to the symptoms associated with the illness.

Symptoms Associated with CFS

Upper Respiratory Tract Illnesses

As discussed in Chap. 1, there had been several studies investigating the aetiology of chronic fatigue throughout its medical history. One factor that had been repeatedly explored was the possible role of viral infections. For example, Straus et al. (1985) focussed on the EBV in the syndrome's aetiology (Straus et al., 1985). Although no causative link was found, it was suggested that patients with CFS were more susceptible to upper respiratory tract infections (URTIs) and that these might be exacerbating their symptoms.

In order to examine this more closely, we conducted a study investigating the link between CFS and URTIs (Smith, Thomas, Borysiewicz, & Llewelyn, 1999). Results of this self-report diary study indicated that patients with CFS reported more URTIs, more severe symptoms and greater use of medication for these illnesses than a healthy control group over a 10-week period. Although of note, this was a subjective study and required replication using appropriate virologic techniques.

In 2015, we reported a study that aimed to replicate and extend this study using a more rigorous research design and methodology (Smith & Thomas, 2015). In this multidisciplinary perspective study, the incidence of URTIs was again investigated in a diary study but also included objective measures of illness severity. These measures included nasal secretion and sub-lingual temperature together with virus isolation from nasal swabs and antibody changes. The study replicated previous findings that patients with CFS more frequently report upper respiratory virus infections than the healthy control group. More importantly, however, was that the virology data suggested that this was not due to a reporting bias but reflected greater susceptibility to infection.

The following sections will discuss findings from two studies: (1) Thomas and Smith (2006) and (2) Thomas and Smith (2008) which investigated the symptoms associated with CFS. As mentioned in the previous section, our study sample included data from 307 patients with CFS and 126 healthy individuals (control group). Table 2.1 describes the demographic data for the two sample groups.

Table 2.1 Demographic data for the CFS and control groups

	CFS (N = 307)	Controls (N = 126)	F (or χ^2), df, p
Male:Female	30:70	34:66	n/s
Age (s.d.)	42.09 (0.67)	40.88 (1.18)	n/s
Marital status: Married (%)	64.6	50.8	n/s
Educational status: Degree level (%)	17.3	16.7	n/s
Employment status: Employed (%)	32.4	50.0	24.34, 5, 0.001
Social classification: Skilled manual (%)	6.6	13.2	11.69, 5, 0.039

Adapted from Thomas and Smith (2008)

Table 2.2 Frequency of symptoms reported from the symptom checklist

Symptom	%	Symptom	%
Lack of concentration	91	Sore throat	52
Muscle pain	89	Wind	49
Excessive fatigue	87	Insomnia	47
Physical weakness	81	Nausea	46
Legs feeling heavy	80	Shivering	45
Fever	77	Glands swollen	45
Loss of memory	76	Racing heart	44
Headache	70	Chest pain	44
Aching joints	69	Indigestion	41
Sensitivity to noise	59	Panic attacks	40
Bloated stomach	55	Depression	37
Sweating	54	Allergies	35
Sore eyes	53	Earache	33
Sensitivity to light	53		

Adapted from Thomas and Smith (2006)

Individual Symptoms and Illness Severity

A symptoms checklist developed specifically to be administered to patients with CFS presented participants with 28 physical (e.g. *legs feeling heavy*) and psychological ailments (e.g. *anxiety/panic feelings*) from which they could select the individual symptoms they were currently experiencing (Thomas & Smith, 2008). Table 2.2 presents data that clearly provides evidence of the myriad symptoms experienced by these patients and goes some way to explaining why this illness has been so difficult to diagnose by primary care physicians. Indeed, anecdotal evidence from patients in our longitudinal study suggested that, prior to attending the clinic, they only discovered what was not wrong with them (Thomas, 2009). This caused an increasing feeling of frustration for both the patient and the GP caring for them. To further exacerbate the situation, half of the patients sampled experienced fluctuations in symptom severity with no regular daily pattern. Symptoms could be worse in the morning, then in the afternoon and then in the evening over a period of time, resulting in patients experiencing high levels of uncertainty. These findings corroborate the assertion that CFS is a heterogeneous condition— that is to say, that there is a wide variation in how symptoms present in different individuals.

From Table 2.2, we can see that lack of concentration is reported by the largest percentage of patients. This is followed by muscle pain, excessive fatigue (over 50% of the time), physical weakness (over 50% of the time) and legs feeling heavy—all of which are experienced by over 80% of patients. A further eight symptoms are reported by over 50% of the respondents. Each of the 28 items are significantly more likely to be reported in the patients with CFS than the control group (Thomas & Smith, 2008) as is the total number of symptoms reported (Thomas & Smith, 2008). The majority of patients (41%) rated their illness severity on the CSH scale as being 'bad with some recovery'.

On further questioning, increased rest and sleep were the most effective ways of minimising the negative effects of the illness and that exercise, walking, shopping, mental effort and stress were most often linked with an increase of symptom severity (Thomas & Smith, 2008).

Fatigue-related Symptoms

Excessive fatigue is the defining symptom of the illness. As discussed earlier in the chapter, fatigue is a difficult symptom to accurately measure due to its highly subjective nature. In 1993, Ray and colleagues developed a questionnaire to more accurately measure changes in CFS which could be used in conjunction with management protocols (Ray, Weir, Stewart, Millar, & Hyde, 1993). The profile of fatigue-related symptoms (PFRS) is a 54-item self-report measure composed of four subscales: (1) fatigue, (2) emotional distress, (3) cognitive difficulties and (4) somatic symptoms.

We can see from Table 2.3 that the CFS group reported higher emotional distress, fatigue, cognitive difficulties and somatic symptom scores than the control group.

Table 2.3   PFRS scale data for the CFS and control sample

	CFS (N = 307)	Controls (N = 126)	F, df, p
Emotional distress	47.80	32.51	53.56, 1, 426, 0.001
Fatigue	62.90	23.05	679.10, 1, 424, 0.001
Cognitive difficulties	46.89	23.58	226.50, 1, 426, 0.001
Somatic symptoms	53.27	23.51	269.20, 1, 424, 0.001

Adapted from Thomas and Smith (2008)

Sleep

Sleep disorders have frequently been observed in individuals with CFS (e.g. Moldofsky, 1996). Further sleep studies in the course of CFS research have shown that, when compared to a non-CFS group, patients have more difficulty falling asleep and spent less time asleep.

In a subjective assessment of sleep, abnormalities were found to be related to personality and measures of physical and mental health (Smith et al., 1996; Thomas & Smith, 2008). A brief four-item measure of sleep behaviour asked individuals to report how many hours (on average) they slept per night. The remaining three items required them to respond to questions—ranging from never through to very often—about the quality of their sleep (e.g. *how often do you feel rested from your night's sleep?*). Patients with CFS reported feeling significantly less rested by sleep than healthy controls (CFS = 18%; controls = 1%: χ^2 = 126.00, df = 4, p < 0.001) even though they reported on average seven hours of sleep per night, a figure comparable to the controls.

Psychopathology and Mood

As indicated in the 28-item checklist, anxiety and depression are included as significant symptoms associated with CFS when compared to a healthy population (Thomas & Smith, 2008). To investigate this further, we administered standardised subjective questionnaire measures for (1) depression (Radloff, 1977), (2) anxiety (Spielberger, Gorsuch, & Lushene, 1971), (3) mood (Smith et al., 1999) and (4) positive and negative affect (Zevon & Tellegen, 1982).

As you can see from Table 2.4, our study showed that the CFS group reported higher levels of anxiety, depression and negative mood together with lower levels of alertness, hedonic tone and positive mood when compared to the control group (Thomas & Smith, 2008).

Table 2.4 Subjective measures of psychopathology and mood for the CFS and control samples

	CFS (N = 307)	Controls (N = 126)	F, df, p
Depression	41.46	35.07	41.58, 1, 424, 0.001
Anxiety	49.36	40.45	55.50, 1, 421, 0.001
Alertness	188.73	290.27	536.70, 1, 431, 0.001
Hedonic tone	122.78	234.17	1227.05, 1, 431, 0.001
Anxiety	74.15	105.29	174.23, 1, 431, 0.001
Positive mood	25.88	36.05	98.16, 1, 424, 0.001
Negative mood	23.95	14.14	71.44, 1, 425, 0.001

Adapted from Thomas and Smith (2008)

Table 2.5 Psychosocial measures for the CFS and control samples

	CFS (N = 307)	Controls (N = 126)	F, df, p
Daily hassles	46.51	32.73	14.26, 1, 421, 0.001
Self-esteem	57.32	58.91	n/s
Perceived stress	26.76	22.55	21.851, 1, 421, 0.001
Positive life events	0.78	1.26	12.65, 1, 426, 0.001
Negative life events	2.34	2.66	n/s

Adapted from Thomas and Smith (2008)

Psychosocial Factors

Psychosocial factors refer to how the combination of psychological and social factors affect an individual's well-being. Here, stress, self-esteem and day-to-day irritations will be discussed along with how individuals with CFS deal with everyday problems.

In order to investigate the psychosocial factors associated with CFS we used standardised measures of (1) daily hassles (Kanner, Coyne, Schaefer, & Lazarus, 1981), (2) self-esteem (Fleming & Watts, 1980), (3) perceived stress (Cohen, Kamarack, & Mermelstein, 1983) and (4) life events (Henderson, Bryne, & Duncan-Jones, 1981).

As you can see from Table 2.5, our study showed that the CFS group reported higher levels of daily hassles and stress, with fewer positive life events than the controls. There was no difference between the groups in terms of self-esteem or negative life events (Thomas & Smith, 2008).

Cognition

There is a plethora of research that has examined the association between fatigue and impairments in cognitive functioning. When considering mental fatigue, deficits in tasks that require focussed attention, speed and accuracy become more pronounced as the person becomes increasingly fatigued. This has been demonstrated in studies of healthy, sleep-deprived individuals (Smith et al., 1993). Investigations into physical fatigue had indicated that impairments occur in simple and choice reaction time tasks (LaManca et al., 1998).

In CFS research, impairments in motor speed, sustained attention and speed of cognitive processing are often present (e.g. Smith et al., 1996) together with deficits in verbal and non-verbal memory tasks (Marshall et al., 1996; Marcel, Komaroff, Faioli, Kornish, & Albert, 1996; Short, McCabe, & Tooley, 2002).

However, a review of the literature by Fry and Martin (1996) uncovered discrepancies between reports of objective measures of cognitive impairment and subjective measures of cognitive failures. They concluded that patients' perceived level of impairment appeared much higher than the objectively measured data suggested. These data may, however, be explained by the cognitive tasks chosen not being suitable to measure the impairments associated with CFS (Wearden & Appleby, 1996) and/or the small number of individuals studied (i.e. poor experimental power).

To address this, both subjective questionnaire and objective computerised measures were used to investigate cognition in CFS. In addition, factors significantly associated with poorer performance such as demographic data, pre-morbid intelligence, illness severity, psychopathology, psychosocial factors and sleep data were accounted for in the data analysis (Thomas & Smith, 2008).

For subjectively measuring cognition, we used the cognitive failures questionnaire (CFQ; Broadbent, Cooper, Fitzgerald, & Parkes, 1982) and the objective measures included a battery of cognitive performance tasks including (1) immediate recall—which provides information about deficits in short-term memory, (2) variable fore-period simple reaction time—which provides information about impairments in motor speed, (3) repeated digits—which provides information about levels of vigilance and (4) the Stroop colour-word interference task—which taps into inhibitory processing (Stroop, 1935). The CFQ measures failures in perception, memory and motor function and asks individuals to rate how often certain

Table 2.6   Objective measures of cognitive performance

	CFS (N = 307)	Controls (N = 126)	F, df, p
Episodic memory	6.1	7.5	$F(1, 430) = 39.92, p < 0.001$
Vigilance	11.2	13.8	$F(1, 383) = 26.80, p < 0.001$
Motor speed	481.1	284.1	$F(1, 430) = 34.30, p < 0.001$
Word/colour interference	113.5	85.9	$F(1, 427) = 52.68, p < 0.001$

Adapted from Thomas and Smith (2008)

things happened over the past six months (e.g. *how often do you bump into people?*). Each of these measures were used as they corresponded to the impairments that patients with CFS had reported.

As we can see from Table 2.6, the CFS group performed significantly worse than the controls for each of the cognitive tasks recalling fewer words, recording slower reaction times, lower levels of vigilance and performing more slowly on the interference task. The CFS group also reported more cognitive difficulties on the CFQ (CFS = 60.53; control = 38.35; $F(1, 419) = 156.00, p < 0.001$) than the control group (Thomas & Smith, 2008).

SUMMARY

The aim of the studies outlined above (Thomas & Smith, 2006, 2008) was to investigate the impairments associated with CFS in line with the Guidelines for Research (Sharpe et al., 1991). In order to address the heterogeneity of CFS, we recruited a large cohort of patients fitting the CDC criteria (Fukuda et al., 1994). In order to provide a suitable comparison group, we recruited demographically matched healthy controls and administered the same measures to both groups. In addition, we collected follow-up data on the CFS cohort in order to chart the natural progression of the illness over time. In terms of recovery, we found that prognosis in the untreated illness was poor. This, together with the significant impact that the syndrome has on an individual's day-to-day functioning and the increased uptake of healthcare resources by patients, led to urgent calls for the development of interventions for CFS. The impact of the illness on daily functioning was confirmed by the numerous individual physical and mental symptoms reported by those participating in our research. Problems with sleep quality and the presence of comorbid mood disorder were also identified together with lower levels of alertness and hedonic tone and higher levels of anxiety.

Of particular importance was that we were able to identify and measure the cognitive impairments associated with CFS using performance tasks. This included deficits in memory, motor speed, vigilance and inhibitory processing. This was the first time that a research group had reported such deficits objectively and was a robust finding due to the fact they had addressed the methodological flaws from previous research. We had, therefore, developed a package of subject and objective measures that could be used to investigate the efficacy of future interventions for CFS.

When we consider the biopsychosocial model in relation to CFS, we have provided evidence of (1) an increased susceptibility to URTIs (biological factors), (2) impairments in emotional distress, cognitive failures and cognitive performance (psychological factors) and (3) increased levels of perceived stress, daily hassles and difficulties in dealing with everyday problems (interpersonal factors). Further interpersonal factors such as communication between patient and clinician and circumstantial factors such as influence of healthcare policies will be covered in Chap. 3, Healthcare provision for CFS.

REFERENCES

Afari, N., & Buchwald, D. (2003). Chronic fatigue syndrome: A review. *American Journal of Psychiatry, 160*, 221–236.

Andersen, M. M., Permin, I. H., & Albrecht, F. (2004). Illness and disability in Danish chronic fatigue syndrome patients at diagnosis and 5-year follow up. *Journal of Psychosomatic Research, 56*, 217–229.

Broadbent, D. E., Cooper, P. F., Fitzgerald, P., & Parkes, K. R. (1982). The Cognitive Failures Questionnaire (CFQ) and its correlates. *British Journal of Clinical Psychology, 21*, 1–16.

Cairns, R., & Hotopf, M. (2005). A systematic review describing the prognosis of Chronic Fatigue Syndrome. *Occupational Medicine, 55*, 20–31.

Cohen, S., Kamarack, T., & Mermelstein, R. (1983). A global measure of perceived stress. *Journal of Health and Social Behaviour, 24*, 385–396.

Engel, G. L. (1980). The clinical application of the biopsychosocial model. *American Journal of Psychiatry, 137*, 535–544.

Fleming, J. S., & Watts, W. A. (1980). The dimensionality of self-esteem: Some results from a college sample. *Journal of Personality and Social Psychology, 39*, 21–29.

Fry, A. M., & Martin, M. (1996). Fatigue in the Chronic Fatigue Syndrome: A cognitive phenomenon? *Journal of Psychosomatic Research, 41*, 415–426.

Fukuda, K., Straus, S., Hickie, I., Sharpe, M. C., Dobbins, J. G., Komaroff, A., et al. (1994). The Chronic Fatigue Syndrome: A comprehensive approach to its definition and study. *Annals Internal Medicine, 121,* 953–959.

Henderson, S., Bryne, D. G., & Duncan-Jones, P. (1981). *Neurosis and the social environment.* Sydney, Australia: Academic Press.

Holmes, G. P., Kaplan, J. E., Gantz, N. M., Komaroff, A. L., Schonberger, L. B., Straus, S. E., et al. (1988). CFS: A working case definition. *Annals Internal Medicine, 108,* 387–389.

Kanner, A. D., Coyne, J. C., Schaefer, C., & Lazarus, R. S. (1981). Comparison of two modes of stress measurement: Minor daily hassles and uplifts versus major life events. *Journal of Behavioural Medicine, 4,* 1–39.

LaManca, J. J., Sisto, S. A., DeLuca, J., Johnson, S. K., Lange, G., Pareja, J., et al. (1998). Influence of exhaustive treadmill exercise on cognitive functioning in Chronic Fatigue Syndrome. *American Journal of Medicine, 105,* 59S–65S.

Marcel, B., Komaroff, A. J., Faioli, L. R., Kornish, R. J., & Albert, M. S. (1996). Cognitive deficits in patients with CFS. *Biological Psychiatry, 40,* 535–541.

Marshall, P. S., Watson, D., Steinberg, P., Cornblatt, B., Peterson, P. K., Callies, A., et al. (1996). An assessment of cognitive function and mood in CFS. *Biological Psychiatry, 39,* 199–206.

Moldofsky, H. (1996). Fibromyalgia, sleep disorder and Chronic Fatigue Syndrome. In *Chronic Fatigue Syndrome* (Ciba Foundation Symposium 173) (pp. 262–279). Chichester: Wiley.

Nisenbaum, R., Jones, A. B., Jones, J. F., & Reeves, W. C. (2000). Longitudinal analysis of symptoms reported by patients with CFS. *Annals of Epidemiology, 10,* 458.

Price, R. K., North, C. S., Wessely, S., & Fraser, V. J. (1992). Estimating the prevalence of CFS and associated symptoms in the community. *Public Health Report, 107,* 514–522.

Radloff, L. S. (1977). The CES-D scale: A self-report depression scale for research in the general population. *Applied Psychology Measure, 1,* 385–401.

Ranjith, G. (2005). Epidemiology of Chronic Fatigue Syndrome. *Occupational Medicine, 55,* 13–19.

Ray, C., Weir, W. R. C., Stewart, D., Millar, P., & Hyde, G. (1993). Ways of coping with CFS: Development of an illness management questionnaire. *Social Science and Medicine, 37,* 385–391.

Reyes, M., Dobbins, J. G., Nisenbaum, R., Subedar, N. S., Randall, B., & Reeves, W. C. (1999). CFS progression and self-defined recovery: Evidence from the CDC surveillance system. *Journal of Chronic Fatigue Syndrome, 5,* 17–27.

Reynolds, K. J., Vernon, S. D., Bouchery, E., & Reeves, W. C. (2004). The economic impact of Chronic Fatigue Syndrome. *Cost Effectiveness and Resource Allocation, 2,* 4.

Russo, J., Katon, W., Clark, M., Kith, P., Sintay, M., & Buchwald, D. (1998). Longitudinal changes associated with improvements in CFS patients. *Journal of Psychosomatic Research, 45,* 67–76.

Sharpe, M. C., Archard, L. C., Banatvala, J. E., Borysiewicz, L. K., Clare, A. W., David, A., et al. (1991). CFS: Guidelines for research. *Journal of the Royal Society of Medicine, 84,* 118–121.

Short, K., McCabe, M., & Tooley, G. (2002). Cognitive functioning in CFS and the role of depression, anxiety and fatigue. *Journal of Psychosomatic Research, 52,* 475–483.

Smith, A. P., Borysiewicz, L., Pollock, J., Thomas, M., Perry, K., & Llewelyn, M. (1999). Acute fatigue in Chronic Fatigue Syndrome. *Psychological Medicine, 29,* 283–290.

Smith, A. P., Brockman, P., Flynn, R., Maben, A., & Thomas, M. (1993). An investigation of the effects of coffee on alertness and performance during the day and night. *Neuropsychobiology, 27,* 217–233.

Smith, A., Pollock, J., Thomas, M., Llewelyn, M., & Borysiewicz, L. (1996). The relationship between subjective ratings of sleep and mental functioning in healthy subjects and patients with chronic fatigue syndrome. *Human Psychopharmacology, 11,* 161–167.

Smith, A., Thomas, M., Borysiewicz, L., & Llewelyn, M. (1999). Chronic fatigue syndrome and susceptibility to upper respiratory tract infections. *British Journal of Health Psychology, 4,* 327–335.

Smith, A., & Thomas, M. (2015). Chronic fatigue syndrome and increased susceptibility to upper respiratory tract infections and illnesses. *Fatigue: Biomedicine, Health & Behaviour, 3,* 156–163.

Spielberger, C., Gorsuch, R., & Lushene, R. E. (1971). *STAI manual for the state-trait anxiety inventory.* Palo Alto, CA: Consulting Psychologists Press.

Straus, S., Tosato, G., Armstrong, G., Lawley, T., Preble, O. T., Henle, W., et al. (1985). Persisting illness and fatigue in adults with evidence of Epstein-Barr virus infection. *Annals of Internal Medicine, 102,* 7–16.

Stroop, J. R. (1935). Studies of interference in serial verbal reactions. *Journal of Experimental Psychology, 18,* 643–662.

Thomas, M. (2009). *Exploring the beliefs and underlying functional deficits associated with CFS and the identification of predictors of recovery and successful illness management.* PhD thesis, University of Wales.

Thomas, M., & Smith, A. (2006). An investigation of the long-term benefits of antidepressant medication in the recovery of patients with Chronic Fatigue Syndrome. *Human Psychopharmacology, 21,* 503–509.

Thomas, M., & Smith, A. (2008). An investigation into the cognitive deficits associated with Chronic Fatigue Syndrome. *Open Neurology Journal, 2,* 78–88.

Wearden, A. J., & Appleby, L. (1996). Research on cognitive complaints and cognitive functioning in patients with Chronic Fatigue Syndrome: What conclusions can we draw? *Journal of Psychosomatic Research, 41,* 197–211.

Zevon, M. A., & Tellegen, A. (1982). The structure of mood change: An idiographic/nomothetic analysis. *Journal of Personality and Social Psychology, 43,* 111–122.

CHAPTER 3

Healthcare Provision for Chronic Fatigue Syndrome

Abstract This chapter focuses on healthcare provision for people with CFS in line with recommendations made by the CMO and the CFS/ME Working Group. The chapter begins with a survey of patient and GP illness beliefs and goes on to discuss the efficacy of pharmacological therapies. Finally, the chapter presents outcomes of three behavioural therapies used to manage symptoms of the illness. These include multi-convergent therapy developed by a physiotherapist and the counselling services and rehabilitation courses run by Action for ME. The efficacy of these therapies was evaluated using the subjective and objective developed in previous research.

Keywords Chronic fatigue syndrome • Multi-convergent therapy • Counselling • Rehabilitation course • Intervention

In the previous chapters we discussed three pivotal reports which aimed at bringing consensus between clinicians and researchers in the UK regarding the definition, symptomology and possible interventions for chronic fatigue syndrome (CFS). The Oxford Guidelines for Research acted to facilitate comparability between studies and to recommend ways in which research could develop (Sharpe et al., 1991). The Royal Colleges report recommended that all clinicians accept the existence of the illness stating that, 'No patient should feel that their credibility is being doubted. There is no place

© The Author(s) 2018
M. Thomas, *"Tired all the Time"*,
https://doi.org/10.1007/978-3-319-93913-1_3

in the clinical consultation for such statements as "there is nothing wrong with you" or "it is all in the mind", just as there is no place for such statement as "you have ME—there is nothing I can do"' (Wessely, 1996, p. 501). In addition, the report urged practitioners to provide a service for patients and take steps to manage patients in their care (Royal Colleges of Physicians, Psychiatrists and General Practitioners, 1996). The CFS/ME Working Group recommended that cognitive behaviour therapy (CBT) and graded exercise were the most successful methods for managing symptoms of the illness (CFS/ME Working Group, 2002).

The National Institute for Health and Care Excellence (NICE) provides national guidance and advice to improve health and social care (www.nice.org.uk). NICE published guidance for patients with CFS, carers and service providers in 2007 (CFS/ME: diagnosis and management clinical guideline [CG53]). The guidelines advised that a diagnosis should be made following the exclusion of other conditions for which fatigue is a primary symptom. It recommends that these symptoms should have persisted for four months and that healthcare professionals should encourage cautious optimism in terms of outcomes whilst providing realistic and honest information to patients. CBT, graded exercise therapy (GET) and activity management programmes are recommended in an individualised, patient-centred programme which should also include addressing sleep hygiene and physical, emotional and cognitive symptoms (www.nice.org.uk). The NICE guidelines for CFS are due to be reviewed during 2018.

Each of the guidelines acknowledge the role of GPs as gatekeepers to healthcare services and the importance of patients feeling that they were being believed by clinicians. Indeed, anecdotal accounts from the CFS outpatient clinic uncovered a pattern of the interviews between patients and their GPs took when the illness first began manifesting itself. When first presenting to primary care, patients reported that the doctor would carry out physical examinations and a variety of blood tests. When the test results came back as unremarkable, some GPs began to insist that 'there is nothing wrong with you'. Others reported that they were told to 'pull themselves together' or 'just go out and enjoy yourself, try to forget about it'. These scenarios expressing doubt about the existence of the illness arising from a lack of awareness of specialised knowledge often led to a breakdown in any previous relationship there might have been between patient and doctor (Thomas, 2009).

In order to quantify these anecdotal claims, we conducted a survey of primary healthcare provision to gauge both patients with CFS and GPs beliefs (Thomas & Smith, 2005).

SURVEY OF PRIMARY HEALTHCARE PROVISION

There had been several surveys conducted to elicit the views of patients and clinicians about the diagnosis and management of CFS. For example, Deale and Wessely (2001) surveyed patients' opinions of medical care in the UK. There had, however, been more studies looking at physicians' perceptions including a national UK survey conducted by Campion in 2004 and an Australian survey conducted by Steven in 2000.

The patient survey involved 68 patients with CFS who had been referred to a specialised clinic which asked them to rate their satisfaction with the medical care offered at the clinic (Deale & Wessely, 2001). Only one-third of the patients reported being satisfied with the quality of the care they received during their illness. The remaining two-thirds reported that delay, dispute or confusion over diagnoses were the root causes of their dissatisfaction and many had previously rejected a psychiatric diagnosis. The patients who were satisfied with the care provided said their doctors had empathy and were supportive. This was in direct contrast to those who were dissatisfied. In fact, empathy and support were felt to be of greater importance even in cases where the GP had admitted lacking in knowledge about the illness. These findings confirm the value of effective communication between doctor and patient in dealing with CFS.

A lack of advice and support from clinicians can lead to individuals looking for other, less reliable, sources of information. In an Australian survey by Kisely (2002), 225 websites directed at individuals with CFS were reviewed over a two-week period. Although it was found that there was a range of information provided about the treatment, there was general agreement that graded exercise and avoiding prolonged rest were the best management strategies. Most sites reviewed (64%) attributed the advice on the site to a named author but only 25–30% recommended that readers clarify any information offered with a healthcare professional, or more worryingly avoided the inclusion of inaccurate statements (Kisely, 2002).

In 2003, Åsbring and Närvänen conducted semi-structured interviews with 26 physicians, all of whom had working knowledge of CFS or fibromyalgia (FM). FM—sometimes called fibromyalgia syndrome (FMS)—is a chronic condition where pain all over the body is a major problem. Additional symptoms include chronic fatigue, sleep abnormalities, muscle stiffness and problems with concentration and memory. Due to the overlapping nature of the symptoms experienced by individuals with CFS and FM, some researchers have studied these conditions in tandem. Åsbring and Närvänen found that physicians were concerned that their lack of specialist knowledge was preventing them from providing appropriate healthcare support for their patients and, therefore, led to their role being questioned by the patient. There was also a feeling that some clinicians viewed CFS as a less serious illness when compared to those with 'disease status' and, worse still, were sceptical about the illness' existence. These views have been supported by further studies such as Steven's GP survey (2000) and the UK survey conducted by Campion (2004). In the Campion survey, 300 questionnaires were sent out to GP surgeries in ten Health Authorities in England, Scotland and Wales. Five of the authorities surveyed had specialised centres for CFS and were matched with five that did not. One conclusion from the study was that GPs in areas with specialised CFS provision were more likely to believe that the condition existed but that they were not more inclined to diagnose the illness than those in areas without specialised services. This suggests that there was limited flow of specialist knowledge from the centres to GP surgeries (Campion, 2004).

In order to investigate this topic further, we conducted a survey of GPs from a single health authority in Wales and with patients recruited to our CFS patient panel to see if the situation had changed following the recommendations made in the report by the Royal Colleges in 1996 (CFS/ME Joint Working Group) and a report by the National Task Force in 1998 (National Task Force on CFS/ME, 1998) (Thomas & Smith, 2005). The GPs were contacted via the official postbags for the area's practices. Two short questionnaire booklets were developed to collect as much comparable data between the patients and GPs as possible.

Ninety-two patient survey questionnaires were completed and returned (48% response rate) and 43 GP surveys were returned (39% response rate). Although the response rates were relatively low, they were comparable with similar surveys of patients (Cooper, 2000) and GPs (Steven, 2000). We could, therefore, put forward the view that these data do represent an accurate portrayal of patient and GP opinions as long as it is discussed in relation to the situation in Wales.

Of the 92 patient respondents, 84.8% reported that they still had CFS—indicating a 15.2% recovery rate—and the average illness duration for the group was 13 years. When asked to rate their illness severity using the CSH scale (Thomas & Smith, 2008), over 60% of the patients reported feeling 'bad with some recovery' or were 'recovering with occasional relapses'. Just over 50% of the sample had received a diagnosis from their GP taking, on average, 6.58 appointments to do so. Over half of the patients (52.6%) thought that they had CFS before the GP diagnosed the illness. When asked where they obtained additional information about CFS 52.2% said the ME Association, but 63% turned to friends or colleagues with CFS and newspaper or magazine articles for information.

The majority of the patient sample (82.6%) reported that their GP had conducted investigative tests to exclude other conditions including (1) a full range of blood tests (90.9%), (2) a test for the Epstein-Barr virus (EBV) (51.9%) and (3) tests for other viral infections (48.1%). Additional investigations including thyroid function tests, hormone function tests, rheumatoid factor tests, ECG, lung function tests and MRI scans were also reported.

Over half of the patients (59.8%) had been offered symptom management strategies by their GP. The most frequent of these was antidepressant therapy (92.7%) or analgesics—not including 'over-the-counter' medicines (36.4%). Other management strategies offered included CBT, GET, occupational therapy (OT) and counselling. Thirty-three patients were referred to secondary care, attending a range of outpatient departments including general medicine (16), cardio/thoracic (3), psychological medicine (3), immunology (2), dentistry (1), ear nose and throat (1), neurology (1) and virology (1). Two patients attended homeopathy clinics and another received a private consultation. A large number (77.2%) turned to alternative therapies to alleviate their symptoms—spending on average £981, with one person reporting spending as much as £7000 on alternative therapies.

Moving on to the GP survey, 55.8% believed that the condition called CFS existed and of these 67.4% had made a diagnosis taking, on average, 6.2 separate appointments to do so. None of the GPs reported using recognised criteria for CFS—such as the Oxford (Sharpe et al., 1991) or CDC (Fukuda et al., 1994), preferring to either conduct investigative tests to rule out other illness (68.8%) and/or refer on to secondary care.

Of the subgroup of GPs who reported diagnosing CFS, 89.3% offered treatment strategies to the patient. The majority of GPs prescribed antidepressant therapy to patients with CFS—the most common (84%) being selective serotonin re-uptake inhibitors (SSRIs). Other antidepressants prescribed were serotonin/noradrenalin re-uptake inhibitors (SNRI) (28%) and the tricyclic and related antidepressants (24%). None of the GP surgeries had trained nurses, occupational therapists or physiotherapists offering support, advice or treatment to manage patients in the primary care setting. They also reported being unaware of any such services being available in their locality. Just over half of the GPs (56.7%) were aware that there was a consultant in the area who had specialist knowledge of CFS. Other outpatient departments that GPs referred to included general medicine (16.7%), rheumatology (6.7%), neurology (6.7%) and psychological medicine (6.7%).

An interesting finding from our patient survey was their views on the use of medication to manage their symptoms. Pain is often associated with CFS and 20 patients reported that they had been prescribed pain relief to manage their symptoms. Only six of these reported any benefit from taking analgesics—the remainder reporting either no benefit (13) or felt that the medication made their symptoms worse. The most common drugs prescribed by GPs were antidepressants. Fifty-one patients reported taking antidepressant medication to manage their symptoms. Only nine reported that this form of medication improved their symptoms—the remainder reporting either no benefit (22) or felt that the medication made their symptoms worse (18).

In the previous chapter (Chap. 2), a large-scale study charting the natural illness history of 307 patients fitting the Centre for Disease Control and Prevention (CDC) (Fukuda et al., 1994) for CFS over a three-year period was discussed (Thomas & Smith, 2006, 2008). These patients attended an outpatient clinic specifically set up to research CFS in South Wales and agreed to join our participant panel. Each patient was evaluated by means of (1) established subjective measures designed to assess the possible psychopathological, biopsychosocial and psychosocial factors associated with the illness and (2) a battery of objective performance tasks designed to highlight changes in cognition. These measures were compared to 126 matched controls (matched by aged, gender, social status and education) were recruited from the general population (Thomas & Smith, 2008). Subjective measures included fatigue (Ray, Weir, Stewart, Millar, & Hyde, 1993), individual symptoms (Smith, Pollock, Thomas, Llewelyn, & Borysiewicz, 1996), illness severity (Smith et al., 1996), sleep quality (Smith et al., 1996), anxiety (Spielberger, Gorsuch, & Lushene, 1971), depression (Radloff, 1977), mood (Zevon & Tellegen, 1982; Smith et al., 1996) and stress (Cohen, Kamarack, & Mermelstein, 1983). Objective measures included free recall, motor speed and vigilance tasks (Smith et al., 1996) together with a word/colour interference task (Stroop, 1935). Our research into the wide range of impairments associated with CFS was as a result of the guidance from the Oxford consensus meeting (Sharpe et al., 1991). Our findings demonstrating measurable deficits in CFS (Thomas & Smith, 2008) provided us with a batch of subjective and objective measures which could be used to evaluate the efficacy of possible intervention strategies as they had previously assessed recovery in the untreated illness (Thomas, 2009).

Interventions for CFS have been categorised as behavioural and pharmacological with some groups combining these approaches (Morris et al., 1998). Two behavioural therapies had been shown to be successful in managing symptoms of the illness, namely, CBT and GET (Deale, Chalder, Marks, & Wessely, 1997; Fulcher & White, 1997), and these interventions had been recommended in reports to the chief medical officer (CMO) (Royal Colleges of Physicians, Psychiatrists and General Practitioners, 1996) and by NICE (www.nice.org.uk). In addition, organisations such as Action for ME (AfME) had developed a range of services, including counselling and rehabilitation courses, designed specifically for individuals with CFS which had been reported as being well received by their clients (Harrison, Smith, & Sykes, 2002).

Pharmacological Therapy

Due to the lack of formal management strategies being available together with the complex nature of the illness, possible treatments had, in the past, been investigated on a pragmatic basis. This meant, to a certain extent, studies were conducted that focussed on pharmacological-based treatments aimed at alleviating some of the symptoms associated with CFS (Goodnick, Sandoval, Brickman, & Klimas, 1992; Vercoulen et al., 1996; Hickie, 1999 for example). Co-morbid anxiety and depression together with problems of sleep disturbance (see Chap. 2) became the focus for treatment (O'Malley et al., 1999). Although antidepressant therapy has been shown to be successful in alleviating certain symptoms associated with CFS, there was no firm evidence to suggest that they facilitated recovery. In a review of treatments by Rimes and Chalder (2005), three randomised controlled trials (RCTs) of two antidepressants, the SSRI fluoxetine (Vercoulen et al., 1996) and the monoamine-oxidase inhibitor (MAOI) phenelzine (Natelson et al., 1996) were discussed. Two of the trials did not provide significant results for any of the outcome measures used. A third trial, again using fluoxetine (Wearden et al., 1998), showed modest improvements in the levels of depression but had no effect in alleviating fatigue.

When exploring data from the patients recruited to our research we found that a small proportion (17%) had been prescribed antidepressant medication by their GP prior to their referral to the clinic. Approximately half of those taking antidepressants had been prescribed tricyclics (53%) and the rest SSRIs (47%). It was of interest to investigate the role antidepressant therapy played in subsequent recovery by comparing this subgroup of patients to those who were not taking antidepressant medication in an attempt to provide evidence of the possible efficacy of these agents in the otherwise untreated patient.

Longitudinal data were collected at the initial clinic visit and again 6 months, 18 months and 3 years later. Initially we compared scores on our current state of health (CSH) measure over time (Thomas & Smith, 2006) between those prescribed antidepressants with those who were not. Next, we looked at differences between patients taking tricyclic antidepressants, patients taking SSRI antidepressants and those not taking antidepressants (Thomas & Smith, 2006). Finally, we administered our 28-item symptom checklist (Smith et al., 1996), the Beck Depression Inventory (Beck, Ward, Mendelson, Mock, & Erbough, 1961), the Trait scale of the Spielberger's state-trait anxiety inventory (STAI; Spielberger et al., 1971), the fatigue subscale of the profile of fatigue-related symptoms (PFRS) questionnaire (Ray et al., 1993) and the sleep quality and activity levels questionnaires (Smith et al., 1996). Of the antidepressant subgroup questioned, 61% reported that the medication had been helpful in alleviating their symptoms.

At the initial clinic visit there was no difference between the demographics or the measures outlined above for the patients taking antidepressants and those who were not. It was only during the follow-up period that differences between the two groups emerged.

As we can see in Table 3.1, the patients taking antidepressant medication were more likely to report being 'almost completely recovered' over the follow-up period than those who were not. These findings were corroborated by the total symptom scores of the two groups with the

Table 3.1 CSH 'almost completely recovered' scores for the antidepressant/no antidepressant groups at baseline, 6-month, 18-month, and 3-year follow-up

Current State of health Measure: 'almost completely recovered'	No antidepressant (%)	Antidepressant (%)
Baseline	0.9	0.0
6 months	2.0	10.5
18 months	6.3	15.8
3 years	6.2	29.2

Table 3.2 Individual symptom scores for the antidepressant/no antidepressant groups at 18 months and 3-year follow-up

Symptom	No antidepressant	Antidepressant	$\chi^2, p\ (df = 1)$
18 months			
Physical fatigue	77	55	7.272, $p < 0.008$
Aching joints	73	55	4.507, $p < 0.029$
3 years			
Physical weakness	79	50	8.538, $p < 0.005$
Physical fatigue	75	50	5.873, $p < 0.017$
Aching joints	76	54	4.660, $p < 0.031$

antidepressant group reporting significantly fewer symptoms at 18 months (no antidepressants = 14.67; antidepressants = 12.24: $F(1, 213) = 4.671$, $p < 0.032$) and 3 years (no antidepressants = 15.12; antidepressants = 11.75; $F(1, 119) = 6.281$, $p < 0.014$).

When we consider individual symptoms, the patients taking antidepressants at baseline were significantly less likely to report symptoms such as physical fatigue and aching joints at 18 months and physical weakness, physical fatigue and aching joints at 3-year follow-up (Table 3.2). There was also a marginal difference in the reporting of lack of concentration as a symptom in the antidepressant group at three-year follow-up.

Those taking antidepressants were also more likely to report improvements in the levels of fatigue on the PFRS scale at 6 months (antidepressants = 53.97; no antidepressants = 60.00: $t = 1.97$, $df = 184$, $p < 0.05$) and 3 years (antidepressants = 49.71; no antidepressants = 58.17: $t = 2.03$, $df = 118$, $p < 0.04$). In addition, patients in the antidepressant group were significantly more likely to report improvements in quality of sleep at 6-month (antidepressants = 24%; no antidepressants = 5%: $\chi^2 = 9.89$, $df = 2$, $p < 0.001$) and 3-year follow-up (antidepressants = 29%; no antidepressants = 7%: $\chi^2 = 9.89$, $df = 2$, $p < 0.007$). They also reported higher activity levels than the no antidepressant group (antidepressants = 21%; no antidepressants = 4%: $\chi^2 = 9.89$, $df = 2$, $p < 0.02$).

When we further split the antidepressant group into those taking SSRIs and those taking tricyclics, there was no difference between the antidepressant subgroups and the no antidepressant group at baseline. However, the patients in the SSRI group were significantly more likely to be in employment at baseline than the tricyclic or no antidepressant groups (SSRI = 49%, tricyclic = 15%, no antidepressant = 28%: $\chi^2 = 6.34$, $df = 2$,

$p < 0.04$). There was no difference in illness severity between the three groups at baseline. However, patients in the SSRI group were marginally more likely to be in the 'almost completely recovered' than the tricyclic or no antidepressant group at 6 and 18 months and significantly more likely to have recovered at 3-year follow-up (SSRI = 43%; Tricyclic = 10%; no antidepressant = 6%: χ^2 = 22.07, df = 8, $p < 0.005$).

As we can see in Table 3.3, patients in the tricyclic antidepressant group reported significantly higher total symptom scores than the SSRI group at baseline. The total symptoms scores for both antidepressant groups were decreased at 18-month and 3-year follow-up compared to the no antidepressant group but this was only significant for those in the SSRI group.

We can see in Table 3.4 that is was the SSRI group of patients who were responsible for the decreased reporting of individual symptoms such as physical weakness and fatigue and aching joints at 18 months and 3-year follow-up time points. In addition, results from the fatigue sub-scale of the PFRS questionnaire suggests that there is an improvement in fatigue scores in the SSRI group over time. The SSRI group also reported

Table 3.3 The total symptom scores for the SSRI, tricyclic and no antidepressant groups at baseline, 18 months and 3-year follow-up

Total symptoms	No antidepressant	SSRI	Tricyclic	F, df, p
Baseline	15.84	13.43	17.27	3.063, 2, 272, <0.048
18 months	14.67	10.32	14.16	4.155, 2, 211, <0.017
3 years	15.12	10.93	12.90	3.455, 2, 118, <0.035

Table 3.4 Individual symptom scores (%) for the SSRI, tricyclic and no antidepressant groups at 18 months and 3-year follow-up

Symptom	No antidepressant	SSRI	Tricyclic	χ^2, p (df = 1)
18 months				
Physical weakness	77	42	89	13.652, $p < 0.001$
Physical fatigue	77	37	74	13.799, $p < 0.001$
Aching joints	73	42	68	7.618, $p < 0.022$
3 years				
Physical weakness	79	29	80	16.470, $p < 0.001$
Physical fatigue	75	36	70	9.154, $p < 0.010$
Aching joints	76	43	70	6.788, $p < 0.034$

a significant improvement in sleep quality at 3-year follow-up when compared to the tricyclic and no antidepressant groups (SSRI = 43%; tricyclic = 10%; no antidepressant = 7%: χ^2 = 20.62, df = 4, p < 0.001). Interestingly, this group also reported significantly increased activity levels at 3-year follow-up (SSRI = 29%; tricyclic = 10%; no antidepressant = 4%: χ^2 = 11.50, df = 4, p < 0.02).

There were no differences between any of the groups in terms of co-morbid anxiety and depression at baseline and there were no significant improvements in the psychopathology of these groups over the follow-up period.

BEHAVIOURAL THERAPY

As mentioned previously in this chapter, CBT and GET had, in the absence of a cure, provided the most successful methods for managing symptoms of the illness (CFS/ME Working Group, 1996). This consensus appeared in accordance with results arising from several treatment trials conducted in the UK (Deale et al., 1997; Fulcher & White, 1997; Sharpe, Hawton, & Simkin, 1996). It was also recommended that multidisciplinary teams of healthcare professionals should offer individualised treatment programmes designed to best suit patient needs.

In 1991, a multi-convergent therapy (MCT) clinic was set up to provide a service for patients with a wide range of problems such as tinnitus, vertigo, anxiety, hyperventilation syndrome and irritable bowel syndrome (Shaw et al., 1991; Sadlier & Stephens, 1995). As the symptoms experienced by patients with these conditions are also sometimes reported in CFS, it was judged that MCT might be of benefit to this patient group. In a retrospective study of 20 patients with CFS treated by this multi-convergent approach, a significant number of patients reported feeling 'better' or 'much better' following the therapy (Sadlier, Evans, Phillips, & Broad, 2000). To provide a more robust evaluation of the therapy, we conducted a randomised, controlled trial comparing MCT to relaxation therapy and a group of patients receiving normal medical care (Thomas et al., 2006, 2008).

Multi-convergent Therapy

MCT employs CBT and GET together with other appropriate strategies in a holistic approach in order to improve sleep quality and to manage any co-morbid mood disturbance. The CBT phase of MCT aimed to (1) identify factors that can influence, precipitate or prolong the illness and (2) improve sleep quality. During this phase of the intervention, dysfunctional beliefs and thought patterns were explored and positive beliefs, thoughts and behaviours re-enforced. During the graded exercise phase of MCT the therapist introduced a programme of planned activity and rest (referred to as 'pacing'). This non-prescriptive graded exercise phase was only introduced after the patient had explored the relationship between fatigue and cognition. The rationale for this aspect of the therapy was based upon a model suggested by Noakes and colleagues where gentle walking was introduced every second day at a level appropriate for each individual case in order to prevent post-exertional malaise (Noakes, St Clair Gibson, & Lambert, 2005). The distance and time walked were increased as the patient's confidence in the belief that this would not cause a relapse of their symptoms grew. The patients were responsible for increasing the level of exercise and providing feedback at the therapy sessions. Mindfulness (or insight) meditation techniques were also blended with the CBT and graded exercise phases. Here, patients were encouraged to fix their thoughts on the present without being distracted by the associations attached to those thoughts or sensations, such as fatigue or pain. This resulted in the individual's ability to reduce the suffering that was associated with physical somatic disorders (Mason & Hargreaves, 2001; Carlson, Speca, Patel, & Goodey, 2004; Grossman, Niemann, Schmidt, & Walach, 2004). Patients could then, in the future, employ this technique when they experience times associated with heightened awareness of pain or fatigue, such as during exercise. In addition, this technique could be used to reduce any intrusive thought patterns experienced at night that prevent the patient from falling asleep (Kabat-Zinn, Lipworth, & Burney, 1985). This process had already been successfully used in conditions associated with pain, immune function, sports and cardiopulmonary function (Sadlier & Stephens, 1995; Davidson et al., 2003; Solberg, Berglund, Engen, Ekeberg, & Loeb, 1996; Shah, Joshi, Mehrotra, Potdar, & Dhar, 2001). Heart rate monitors were used during the sessions to act as a symbol of fitness and wellness, to help prevent vulnerable patients from deteriorating into a 'boom-and-bust' scenario, and to assess the relaxation response (Kabat-Zinn et al., 1985). The monitors enabled the identification of the average peak heart rate for each patient whilst exercising at a sustainable level and to establish cardiac rhythm but were not used to promote exercise. The therapy simultaneously combined facets of behavioural and sometimes pharmacological therapy with fitness training in an attempt to address the many coexisting clinical features of the condition. This multidimensional approach also used aspects of behaviour modification, breathing and relaxation techniques, connective tissue massage and psychodynamic counselling. In addition, all phases of the technique could be delivered by a single therapist in a programme tailored to the individual patient.

As a comparison intervention we used a relaxation procedure based on the work of Ost (1987). This rapid relaxation technique had proved successful for alleviating symptoms in a wide range of problems such as tinnitus and pain as well as CFS (Ost, 1987). The aim of rapid relaxation was to help patients to target specific areas of the illness, thus facilitating symptom relief and offers the patient a way of coping with and managing their symptoms. The therapist guided the patient through the relaxation technique over a period of ten weeks, with each session revising the previous session before moving on to a different major muscle group. Relaxation therapy had been favoured by various centres and patient groups (e.g. AfME) throughout England, Scotland and Wales, and had been used as a comparison by other research groups (Deale et al., 1997). Both the MCT and relaxation therapy sessions were conducted on a one-to-one basis.

The outcome measures used to assess the efficacy of MCT included those described previously (Thomas & Smith, 2008) and, in order to make direct comparisons with other studies (Sharpe et al., 1996, for example), the Karnofsky performance scale (Karnofsky, Abelmann, Craver, & Burchenal, 1948), illness severity and treatment satisfaction measures (Deale et al., 1997) together with global measures of health (Ware & Sherbourne, 1992) were also included. Outcome measure data were collected at baseline, immediately post-therapy and six months post-therapy. There was no difference between the three trial groups in terms of demographics, length of illness, illness severity or Karnofsky performance scores (Karnofsky et al., 1948) at baseline.

In our study (Thomas et al., 2006) we found that the MCT group reported improvements in the following mood and performance measures immediately post-therapy: (1) higher alertness levels (MCT = 233.9; relax = 176.1; control = 170.1: $F(2, 31) = 3.31$, $p < 0.05$) and (2) faster responses on the simple reaction time task (MCT = 375.2 msec; relax = 406.1 msec; control = 441.0 msec: $t = 2.845$, $df = 11$, $p < 0.016$). The MCT group also reported improved sleep quality (MCT = 83.3%; relax = 28.6%; control = 11.1%: $\chi^2 = 14.222$, $df = 4$, $p < 0.007$) post-therapy. When considering illness severity, the MCT group reported greater improvements in (1) health status (MCT = 83.3%; relax = 50.0%; control = 22.2%: χ^2 = 9.78, df = 4, p < 0.044) and (2) activity levels (MCT = 100%; relax = 21.4%; control = 42.9: χ^2 = 29.670, df = 4, p < 0.001). This was accompanied by lower total symptom scores in the MCT group (MCT = 10.42; relax = 14.71; control = 13.78: $F(2, 31)$ = 4.627, p < 0.017).

Using a global assessment of function and satisfaction with treatment post-therapy we found that the MCT group reported (1) greater improvement in their overall condition (MCT = 91.7%; relaxation = 64.3%; control = 22.2%: χ^2 = 13.637, df = 4, p < 0.009), (2) lower levels of fatigue (MCT = 83.3%; relaxation = 57.1%; control = 11.1%: χ^2 = 20.652, df = 4, p < 0.001) and (3) a reduction in disability (MCT = 75%; relaxation = 49.2%; control = 11.1%: χ^2 = 9.699, df = 4, p < 0.046).

Of importance was encouraging data indicating that improvements in the MCT group continued at the six-month follow-up period including (1) higher alertness and faster mean reaction time, (2) improvements in global measures of health, such as overall improvement in their condition, (3) lower fatigue levels and (4) feeling far less impaired by their illness. In terms of acceptability, the MCT group found the therapy useful and were satisfied with it. With regard to the attainment of a Karnofsky performance score of 80% or more (consultant-rated), the MCT group were more likely to meet the desired outcome (MCT = 83.3%; relaxation = 21.4%; control = 0: χ^2 = 17.77, df = 2, p < 0.001). These findings were corroborated by the patient-rated score (Thomas et al., 2006, 2008).

It is important to also discuss the efficacy of relaxation therapy as a strategy for managing fatigue. When we consider the CSH measure, 50% of the relaxation group reported improvements in illness severity following the therapy (Thomas et al., 2006). This finding was corroborated by data from the Karnofsky scale indicating that 50% of these patients reported a 10% improvement in performance (Thomas et al., 2008). In terms of levels of fatigue, 50% of the relaxation group reported that their fatigue was 'much better' or 'very much better' post-therapy. This improvement was maintained six months post-therapy. Although there was no difference in levels of self-report anxiety immediately post-therapy, levels of anxiety were significantly reduced six months post-therapy (t = −3.842, df = 13, p < 0.002). This finding was accompanied by a significant improvement in levels of alertness six months post-therapy (t = −2.500, df = 13, p < 0.027). When considering global measures of health, 64% of the relaxation group reported their coverall condition as 'much better' or 'very much better' post-therapy. This percentage reduced slightly at the six-month follow-up point to 43%. When asked to rate the level of disability caused by CFS, half of this group reported feeling 'much better' or 'very much better' post-therapy and this number was maintained six months later. In terms of acceptability, the relaxation therapy group found the therapy useful and were satisfied with it. We, therefore, found that there were several benefits of relaxation therapy, thus confirming the beliefs of some patient groups that relaxation therapy has a place in alleviating some of the symptoms associated with CFS. Indeed, relaxation therapy is normally a component of the MCT technique and was only omitted from the study to act as the comparison group to evaluate its individual benefits. It is reasonable to suggest that inclusion of relaxation techniques can only enhance the effectiveness of MCT, especially in reducing psychopathology.

Whilst the success of our trial was of note, patients with CFS are well aware that the illness is plagued with bouts of apparent recovery. In these instances, the person can feel as if they have returned to normal health only to be struck down again with the illness weeks or even months later. We believed, therefore, that it would be important to test the robustness of the therapy over a longer time period in a study funded by Healthy Minds at Work. In addition, as the level of illness severity of the participants in the original study was sufficient to prevent them from maintaining employment, it was crucial to assess whether the treatment would facilitate return to the work in this patient group (Smith, Thomas, & Sadlier, 2009).

When considering the Karnofsky performance scores of the MCT group at 3-year follow-up, seven of the nine respondents (77.8%) continued to report function scores of over 70%, indicating normal functioning, five of whom recorded scores in excess of 80%.

As we can see in Table 3.5, only one person reported no improvements in sleep quality or activity levels. There was no significant difference between the total symptom scores at six-month post-therapy and three-year follow-up indicating that those attending MCT sessions continued to report lower total symptom scores over time.

We can see in Table 3.6 that, although the small sample size precludes statistical analysis, patients with MCT appear to be maintaining their six-month post therapy performance levels.

Four of the ten MCT respondents were in employment at the time of this follow-up assessment (two full-time, two part-time) and they had all

Table 3.5 Improvements in activity levels and sleep quality for the MCT participants completing the 3-year follow-up evaluation compared to their baseline
scores

	Pre-therapy level (%) (n)	'Significantly' or 'moderately' increased from pre-therapy (%) (n)
Activity levels	9 (1)	91 (10)
Sleep quality	9 (1)	91 (9)

Table 3.6 Subjective ratings of mood and objective performance data for the
MCT group at six months and three years

Measure	MCT patients (n = 7)	
	Six-months post-therapy	Three-years post-therapy
Mood		
Alertness	205.00	183.85
Hedonic tone	173.57	162.14
Anxiety	76.00	71.43
Episodic memory		
No. of words recalled	10.00	9.00
Simple reaction time		
Mean reaction time	394.25	376.86
Vigilance		
Mean reaction time	777.44	751.80
No. of targets correct	15.57	16.28

returned to their previous employment. Two of the remaining six had
retired due to ill-health. One had since reached state pension age. The
remaining four believed that they were too ill to work.

When exploring the reasons why these patients gave up work, the over-
whelming response was that their previous employment was too emotion-
ally and/or physically demanding. This was also the reason for each not
wishing to return to their previous employment. None of the patients with
MCT blamed their employer's or colleague's attitudes towards CFS for
their reluctance to resume their previous careers. When presented with the
'ideal working conditions' scenario, three agreed that they would now be
able to resume work for a couple of hours per week if a suitable vacancy
and/or training were made available to them. A further participant said
that they would be able to work part-time. The patient who had retired

due to ill-health maintained that even in ideal conditions they would still not be able to work.

We received several complimentary comments from members of the MCT group at three-year follow-up. Typical patient statements include: '*I wish I had received the treatment (MCT) years ago—then I would have not had to leave work*' and '*now I feel that I could maybe do a couple of hours (work) a week*'.

Counselling and Rehabilitation Courses

In 1994, the National Task Force on CFS/post viral fatigue syndrome/ myalgic encephalomyelitis was set up at the request of the Department of Health who had been asked to provide clear guidelines regarding the diagnosis and management of CFS by patient organisations (National Task Force on chronic fatigue syndrome/post viral fatigue syndrome/myalgic encephalitis, 1994). One of these organisations—Westcare UK—played a pivotal role in the task force. Westcare later merged with AfME. One of the remits of the charity was to provide medical services, OT, telephone and face-to-face counselling and residential rehabilitation courses. The aim of these services was to offer coping strategies for their client's illness which include techniques for balancing the levels of activity and rest (sometimes called pacing).

The long-term effectiveness of one of these services, namely the residential rehabilitation courses, had been demonstrated in a preliminary investigation conducted in-house by AfME (Harrison et al., 2002). We were approached by the organisation to conduct a further independent evaluation of their services (Thomas & Smith, 2007).

We used the range of comprehensive subjective measures previously described (Thomas & Smith, 2006, 2008). These were presented as two booklets and (1) administered by AfME at baseline then (2) sent out by our research unit six months later.

In total we recruited 21 residential course clients and 24 counselling clients. There was no difference between the two groups of clients for any of the measures collected at baseline. The caveats being that the mean age of the counselling clients was lower than that of the residential clients (counselling mean age = 39.0; residential mean age = 48.6: $F(1, 43) = 7.651$, $p < 0.008$) and the counselling group consisted on an almost equal male to female split (42:58) compared to the residential clients (14:86) who were predominately female ($\chi^2 = 4.09$, $df = 1$, $p < 0.044$).

We can see in Table 3.7 that the residential course clients reported (1) lower physical and mental fatigue scores, (2) higher positive mood scores and significantly lower negative mood scores and (3) lower levels of depression and emotional distress (PFRS) immediately after completing the course (Thomas & Smith, 2007).

As we can see in Table 3.8, improvements within this group were sustained and further increased at the six-month follow-up point with clients continuing to show the improvements in (1) physical and mental fatigue and (2) lower negative mood scores, depression, anxiety and emotional distress scores. In addition, these clients reported (1) improvements in fatigue, cognitive difficulties, somatic symptom scores and physical symptoms and (2) lower perceived stress and anxiety scores (Thomas & Smith, 2007).

Table 3.7   Residential client questionnaire scores immediately post-course

Measure	Baseline score	Post-course score	t, df, p
Physical fatigue	20.05	12.95	5.203, 18, <0.000
Mental fatigue	13.28	8.56	3.879, 17, <0.001
Depression	49.33	37.22	3.621, 17, <0.002
State anxiety	48.84	39.63	2.704, 18, <0.015
Emotional distress	58.58	43.00	2.871, 18, <0.010

Table 3.8   Residential client questionnaire scores at follow-up

Measure	Baseline score	Follow-up score	t, df, p
Mental health	55.43	65.71	−2.354, 20, <0.029
General health	28.62	42.71	−3.608, 20, <0.002
Physical fatigue	20.29	13.90	5.379, 20, <0.000
Mental fatigue	13.35	10.80	3.243, 19, <0.004
Negative mood	29.45	20.36	4.661, 21, <0.000
Depression	47.57	39.00	3.165, 20, <0.005
Emotional distress	55.09	39.28	3.146, 20, <0.005
Fatigue	66.00	53.50	3.273, 21, <0.004
Cognitive difficulties	50.18	41.45	2.463, 21, <0.023
Somatic symptoms	56.57	46.62	2.115, 20, <0.047
Anxiety	52.62	46.19	3.109, 20, <0.006
Physical symptoms	23.95	20.24	2.610, 20, <0.017
Perceived stress	30.20	26.60	2.882, 19, <0.010

Table 3.9 Counselling client's questionnaire scores at follow-up

Measure	Baseline score	Follow-up score	t, df, p
Mental health	55.48	66.26	−2.908, 22, <0.008
General health	24.54	30.58	−2.204, 23, <0.031
Physical fatigue	19.54	17.08	2.298, 23, <0.031
Mental fatigue	12.88	11.50	2.253, 23, <0.034
Positive mood	22.91	30.27	−2.861, 21, <0.009
Negative mood	27.95	20.50	3.247, 21, <0.004
Depression	46.18	38.82	3.336, 21, <0.003
Emotional distress	51.41	41.59	2.202, 21, <0.039
Fatigue	61.09	51.00	2.805, 21, <0.011
Somatic symptoms	48.82	43.32	2.337, 21, <0.029
Anxiety	50.08	45.46	2.233, 23, <0.036
Physical symptoms	21.74	18.43	2.218, 23, <0.037
Perceived stress	28.46	25.08	2.366, 23, <0.027

As we see in Table 3.9, the counselling clients continued to report improvements at six-month follow-up in (1) physical and mental fatigue and mental and general health scores, (2) positive and negative mood, depression and anxiety and (3) fatigue, somatic symptom and emotional distress. They also reported lower physical symptoms and perceived stress at follow-up.

When we look at the global outcomes at the six-month follow-up point, (1) 83% of the counselling clients and 66% of the residential clients reported that they were 'better' or 'very much better', (2) 67% of the counselling clients and 62% of the residential clients reported that their level of fatigue was 'better' or 'much better', (3) 75% of the counselling clients and 57% of the residential clients reported lower levels of disability, (4) 96% of the counselling clients and 95% of the residential clients were 'satisfied' or 'very satisfied' with the service they had received and (5) 79% of the counselling clients and 86% of the residential clients found the service 'useful' or 'very useful'. Finally, all of the clients who completed our study said that they would recommend the services provided by AfME to other people with CFS (Thomas & Smith, 2007).

Summary

Our patient and GP survey aimed to find out what was being done in primary care to manage patients presenting with CFS primary care in light of the recommendations by the CMO. Patients reported having multiple consultations, firstly with their GP and then in a range of outpatient departments. They were also susceptible to the lure of expensive untested alternative therapies. We found that GPs were not aware of the diagnostic criteria for the condition and that there was no common consensus on how to proceed if CFS was suspected. The most commonly used intervention was antidepressant medication.

In our study looking at the use of antidepressant medication for alleviating the symptoms associated with CFS, we found that there were several important benefits such as a reduction in symptoms and illness severity over a three-year period (Thomas & Smith, 2006). However, due to the fact that the study was retrospective, we did not have any information about how long individuals had been taking this medication before attending the initial clinic visit. In addition, we acknowledge that the antidepressant group were a self-selecting sample. It would be of interest to compare patients prescribed long-term medication with those taking antidepressants for only short periods, and to investigate short-term antidepressant use followed by the long-term monitoring of its effects. In this way it may be possible to offer a more acceptable treatment programme to facilitate recovery in CFS.

In our intervention efficacy studies (Thomas et al., 2006, 2008), we described an holistic, individualised programme: MCT. A trial of the therapy, developed by a physiotherapist, resulted in significant improvements in important aspects of the illness such as illness severity, sleep and levels of activity. Poor sleep and reduced activity had been indicated as confounding factors in perpetuating the illness. Patients also reported feeling significantly more alert after treatment and were less anxious. Of importance were improvements in objective measures of performance in the MCT group in terms of word recall, mean reaction time and increased repeated digits detection in the vigilance task. These findings are unique and important from a treatment point of view. These positive outcomes continued at the six-month follow-up assessment. The efficacy of relaxation was also indicated in our study, especially with regard to reducing psychopathology. This was an important finding as it had already been proposed by patient groups as a method of alleviating the symptoms of CFS and this was the reason why we included a non-intervention control group as a comparison in our trial.

The long-term efficacy of MCT is also indicated. Our three-year follow-up study indicated that patients who attended the therapy continued to maintain the benefits of the intervention reported six-month post-therapy up to three years later (Smith et al., 2009). These included lower levels of fatigue and disability together with improved functioning and illness severity. In addition, the improvements in objective measures of performance were maintained three years later. We also found that MCT had the potential to enable return to work with four of the eight members of the intervention group returning to full- or part-time employment and the remaining four stating that they would work if a suitable job presented itself.

In our evaluation of the services offered by AfME, those attending their rehabilitation course reported significantly lower mental and physical fatigue scores after the course together with improvements in mood and lower anxiety, depression and emotional distress scores. These benefits are sustained and become more wide-ranging over time. Similar positive findings were reported by the clients using the counselling services. These included lower anxiety, depression and perceived stress together with improvements in the number and severity of symptoms, including fatigue and physical symptoms, at the six-month follow-up point. These data were also supported by the global outcome measures with many clients reporting overall improvement in their condition, improved levels of fatigue and reduced levels of disability. The majority of clients rated highly the usefulness of the services, were satisfied with the level of care provided, and would recommend AfME and its services to others with CFS.

REFERENCES

Åsbring, P., & Närvänen, A. (2003). Ideal versus reality: Physicians' perspectives on patients with CFS and Fibromyalgia. *Social Science and Medicine, 57,* 711–720.

Beck, A. T., Ward, C. H., Mendelson, M., Mock, J., & Erbough, J. (1961). An inventory for measuring depression. *Archives of General Psychiatry, 4,* 561–571.

Campion, P. (2004). *National Survey of General Practitioners' beliefs about CFS/ME.* A report to the Linbury Trust.

Carlson, L., Speca, M., Patel, K., & Goodey, E. (2004). Mindfulness-based stress reduction in relation to quality of life, mood, symptoms of stress and levels of cortisol, dehydroepiandrosterone sulphate (DHEAS) and melatonin in breast and prostate cancer outpatients. *Psychoneuroendocrinology, 29,* 448–474.

CFS/ME Joint Working Group. (1996). *A report of a Joint Working Group between the Royal College of Physicians, the Royal College of General Practitioners and the Royal College of Psychiatrists.* London: CFS/ME Joint Working Group.

CFS/ME Working Group. (2002). *Report to the Chief Medical Officer of an independent working group.* London: Department of Health.

Cohen, S., Kamarack, T., & Mermelstein, R. (1983). A global measure of perceived stress. *Journal of Health and Social Behaviour, 24,* 385–396.

Cooper, L. (2000). *Report on survey of local ME group members.* A report in conjunction with Action for ME and ME Association.

Davidson, R., Kabat-Zinn, J., Schumacher, J., Rosenkranz, M., Muller, D., Santorelli, S. F., et al. (2003). Alterations in brain and immune function produced by mindfulness meditation. *Psychosomatatic Medicine, 65,* 564–570.

Deale, A., Chalder, T., Marks, I., & Wessely, S. (1997). Cognitive behaviour therapy for chronic fatigue syndrome: A randomized controlled trial. *American Journal of Psychiatry, 154,* 408–414.

Deale, A., & Wessely, S. (2001). Patients' perceptions of medical care in CFS. *Social Science and Medicine, 52,* 1859–1864.

Fukuda, K., Straus, S., Hickie, I., Sharpe, M. C., Dobbins, J. G., Komaroff, A., et al. (1994). The Chronic Fatigue Syndrome: A comprehensive approach to its definition and study. *Annals of International Medicine, 121,* 953–959.

Fulcher, K. Y., & White, P. D. (1997). Randomised controlled trial of graded exercise in patients with the chronic fatigue syndrome. *British Medical Journal, 314,* 1647–1652.

Goodnick, P. J., Sandoval, R., Brickman, A., & Klimas, N. G. (1992). Bupropion treatment of fluoxetine-resistant chronic fatigue syndrome. *Biological Psychiatry, 32,* 834–838.

Grossman, P., Niemann, L., Schmidt, S., & Walach, H. (2004). Mindfulness-based stress reduction and health benefits: A meta-analysis. *Journal of Psychosomatic Research, 57,* 35–43.

Harrison, S., Smith, A., & Sykes, R. (2002). Residential rehabilitation courses in the self-directed management of Chronic Fatigue Syndrome: A preliminary evaluation. *Journal of Chronic Fatigue Syndrome, 10,* 59–65.

Hickie, I. (1999). Nefazodone for patients with chronic fatigue syndrome. *Australia and New Zealand Journal of Psychiatry, 33,* 278–280.

Kabat-Zinn, J., Lipworth, L., & Burney, R. (1985). The clinical use of mindfulness meditation for the self-regulation of chronic pain. *Journal of Behavioural Medicine, 8,* 163–190.

Karnofsky, D. A., Abelmann, W. H., Craver, L. F., & Burchenal, J. H. (1948). The use of the nitrogen mustards in the palliative treatment of carcinoma. *Cancer, 1,* 634–656.

Kisely, S. (2002). Treatments for CFS and the internet: A systematic survey of what your patients are reading. *Australia and New Zealand Journal of Psychiatry, 36,* 240–245.

Mason, O., & Hargreaves, I. (2001). A qualitative study of mindfulness-based cognitive therapy for depression. *British Journal of Medical Psychology, 74,* 197–212.

Morris, R., Wearden, A., Mullis, R., Strickland, P., Pearson, D. J., Appleby, L., et al. (1998). A double-blind placebo controlled trial of fluoxetine and graded exercise for CFS. *British Journal of Psychiatry, 172,* 485–490.

Natelson, B. H., Cheu, J., Pareja, J., Ellis, S. P., Policastro, T., & Findley, T. W. (1996). Randomised, double-blind, controlled placebo-phase in trial of low-dose phenelzine in the chronic fatigue syndrome. *Psychopharmacology, 124,* 226–230.

National Institute for Health and Care Excellence (NICE). Retrieved March 2018, from www.nice.org.uk

National Task Force on Chronic Fatigue Syndrome/Post Viral Fatigue Syndrome/ Myalgic Encephalitis. (1994). Bristol: Westcare.

National Task Force on CFS/ME. (1998). *NHS services for people with CFS/ME.* Bristol: Westcare.

Noakes, T., St Clair Gibson, A., & Lambert, E. (2005). From catastrophe to complexity: A novel model of integrative central neural regulation of effort and fatigue during exercise in humans: Summary and conclusions. *British Journal of Sports Medicine, 39,* 120–124.

O'Malley, P. G., Jackson, J. L., Santoro, J., Tomkins, G., Balden, E., & Kroenke, K. (1999). Antidepressant therapy for unexplained symptoms and symptom syndromes. *Journal of Family Practice, 48,* 980–990.

Ost, L. (1987). Applied relaxation: Description of a coping technique and review of controlled studies. *Behaviour Research Therapy, 25,* 397–409.

Radloff, L. S. (1977). The CES-D scale: A self-report depression scale for research in the general population. *Applied Psychological Measure, 1,* 385–401.

Ray, C., Weir, W. R. C., Stewart, D., Millar, P., & Hyde, G. (1993). Ways of coping with CFS: Development of an illness management questionnaire. *Social Science and Medicine, 37,* 385–391.

Rimes, K. A., & Chalder, T. (2005). Treatments for chronic fatigue syndrome. *Occupational Medicine, 55,* 32–39.

Royal Colleges of Physicians, Psychiatrists and General Practitioners. (1996). *Chronic Fatigue Syndrome: Report of a joint working group.* London.

Sadlier, M. J., Evans, J. R., Phillips, C., & Broad, A. (2000). A preliminary study into the effectiveness of multi-convergent therapy in the treatment of heterogeneous patients with CFS. *Journal of Chronic Fatigue Syndrome, 7,* 93–100.

Sadlier, M., & Stephens, D. (1995). An approach to the audit of tinnitus management. *Journal of Laryngology and Otology, 109,* 826–829.

Shah, A , Joshi, S., Mehrotra, P., Potdar, N., & Dhar, H. (2001). Effect of Saral meditation on intelligence, performance and cardiopulmonary functions. *The Indian Journal of Medical Science, 55,* 604–608.

Sharpe, M., Archard, L., Banatvala, J., Borysiewicz, L., Clare, A., David, A., et al. (1991). CFS: Guidelines for research. *Journal Royal Society of Medicine, 84,* 118–121.

Sharpe, M., Hawton, K., & Simkin, S. (1996). Cognitive behaviour therapy for Chronic Fatigue Syndrome: A randomised controlled trial. *British Medical Journal, 312,* 22–26.

Shaw, G., Srivastava, E. D., Sadlier, M., Swann, P., James, J. Y., & Rhodes, J. (1991). Stress management for Irritable Bowel Syndrome: A controlled trial. *Digestion, 50,* 36–42.

Smith, A., Pollock, J., Thomas, M., Llewelyn, M., & Borysiewicz, L. (1996). The relationship between subjective ratings of sleep and mental functioning in healthy subjects and patients with chronic fatigue syndrome. *Human Psychopharmocology, 11,* 161–167.

Smith, A., Thomas, M., & Sadlier, M. (2009). Multi-convergent therapy: A possible intervention to aid return to work. *Occupational Health at Work, 6,* 30–32.

Solberg, E., Berglund, K., Engen, O., Ekeberg, O., & Loeb, M. (1996). The effect of meditation on shooting performance. *British Journal of Sports Medicine, 30,* 342–346.

Spielberger, C., Gorsuch, R., & Lushene, R. E. (1971). *STAI manual for the State-trait anxiety inventory.* Palo Alto, CA: Consulting Psychologists Press.

Steven, S. (2000). General Practitioners' beliefs, attitudes and reported actions towards CFS. *Australian Family Physician, 29,* 80–85.

Stroop, J. R. (1935). Studies of interference in serial verbal reactions. *Journal of Experimental Psychology, 18,* 643–662.

Thomas, M. (2009). *Exploring the beliefs and underlying functional deficits associated with CFS and the identification of predictors of recovery and successful illness management.* PhD thesis, University of Wales.

Thomas, M., Sadlier, M., & Smith, A. (2006). The effect of Multi Convergent Therapy on the psychopathology, mood and performance of Chronic Fatigue Syndrome patients: A preliminary study. *Counselling and Psychotherapy Research, 6,* 91–99.

Thomas, M., Sadlier, M., & Smith, A. (2008). A multiconvergent approach to the rehabilitation of patients with chronic fatigue syndrome: A comparative study. *Physiotherapy, 94,* 35–42.

Thomas, M., & Smith, A. (2005). Primary healthcare provision and Chronic Fatigue Syndrome: A survey of patients' and general practitioners' beliefs. *BMC Family Practice, 6,* 49. https://doi.org/10.1186/1471-2296-6-49

Thomas, M., & Smith, A. (2006). An investigation of the long-term effects of antidepressant medication in the recovery of patients with CFS. *Human Psychopharmacology, 21,* 503–509.

Thomas, M., & Smith, A. (2007). The evaluation of counselling and rehabilitation courses for Chronic Fatigue Syndrome patients. *Counselling and Psychotherapy Research, 7*, 164–171.

Thomas, M., & Smith, A. (2008). An investigation into the cognitive deficits associated with Chronic Fatigue Syndrome. *Open Neurology Journal, 2*, 78–88.

Vercoulen, J., Swanink, C. M., Zitman, F. G., Vreden, S. G., Hoofs, M. P., Fennis, J. F., et al. (1996). Randomised, double-blind, placebo-controlled study of fluoxetine in chronic fatigue syndrome. *Lancet, 347*, 1292–1298.

Ware, J. E., & Sherbourne, C. D. (1992). The MOS 36-item short-form health survey (SF-36). *Medical Care, 30*, 473–483.

Wearden, A. J., Morriss, R. K., Mullis, R., Strickland, P., Pearson, D. J., Appleby, L., et al. (1998). Randomised, double-blind, placebo-controlled treatment trial of fluoxetine and graded exercise for chronic fatigue syndrome. *British Journal of Psychiatry, 172*, 485–490.

Wessely, S. (1996). CFS: Summary of a report of a joint committee of the Royal Colleges of Physicians, Psychiatrists and General Practitioners. *Journal of the Royal Colleges of Physicians of London, 30*, 497–504.

Zevon, M. A., & Tellegen, A. (1982). The structure of mood change: An idographic/nomothetic analysis. *Journal of Personality and Social Psychology, 43*, 111–112.

CHAPTER 4

Persistent Fatigue in Chronic Conditions

Abstract This chapter considers fatigue as a secondary but significant symptom in chronic conditions including rheumatoid arthritis, multiple sclerosis, Parkinson's disease and cancer. The chapter describes studies that have investigated the nature of the fatigue experienced in these conditions together with systematic reviews concerning the efficacy of interventions to manage fatigue. Included in this chapter is an in-depth study into the fatigue reported by adults with the neurodevelopmental disorder developmental coordination disorder (DCD). A comparison of the nature of the fatigue in DCD is also compared to that of CFS.

Keywords Chronic conditions • Fatigue • Rheumatoid arthritis • Multiple sclerosis • Parkinson's disease • Cancer • Developmental coordination disorder

In the previous chapters we have discussed the history of chronic fatigue syndrome (CFS), the symptoms associated with the illness and possible interventions. Increasingly over the last ten years patients are reporting persistent and debilitating fatigue as a secondary symptom in a range of chronic diseases. This chapter will provide examples of studies reporting data on the prevalence of fatigue and the problem that it is posing to healthcare providers. It will go on to discuss systematic reviews focussing on the fatigue reported in four chronic conditions, namely rheumatoid arthritis (RA), multiple sclerosis

© The Author(s) 2018
M. Thomas, *"Tired all the Time"*,
https://doi.org/10.1007/978-3-319-93913-1_4

(MS), Parkinson's disease (PD) and cancer. The ways in which fatigue is currently being managed in primary and/or secondary care for these four conditions will also be considered. The chapter will conclude with a study which considers the nature of the fatigue experienced by individuals with developmental coordination disorder (DCD).

In 2015, Nicholson and colleagues highlighted the prevalence and impact of fatigue in Canada's primary care system (Nicholson, Stewart, & Thind, 2015). Their study extracted data on patients reporting the symptom of fatigue together with a non-fatigued comparison group from the Ontario electronic medical records database. Over a one-year period the study reported a prevalence of fatigue at 8.2% and found that these patients made significantly more subsequent visits and received a greater number of medical investigations than the non-fatigued patients. In another study, Cella and colleagues used the patient-reported outcomes measurement information system (PROMIS) fatigue measures to assess a range of chronic conditions over time (Cella et al., 2016). This USA study identified six chronic conditions that present with co-occurring fatigue. These were (1) chronic obstructive pulmonary disease, (2) chronic heart failure, (3) chronic back pain, (4) major depressive disorder, (5) RA and (6) cancer. Their study found that all the above patient groups reported higher levels of fatigue than a general population comparison group and that the severity of fatigue varied across the conditions.

As mentioned at the beginning of the chapter, there are many chronic conditions for which fatigue is a significant symptom. The fatigue experienced in four illnesses will now be considered together as results from systematic reviews of interventions for fatigue in these chronic conditions.

HEALTHCARE PROVISION FOR FATIGUE IN CHRONIC CONDITIONS

Rheumatoid Arthritis

Fatigue is a very common symptom in RA and patients consider it as one of the most important consequences of the disease as it significantly impacts on many aspects of day-to-day functioning. The cause of the fatigue experienced is unknown and it remains unclear as to whether the inflammatory symptoms of RA are associated with fatigue. What is known is that the associated fatigue interacts with the disease process together with cognitive and psychosocial factors. What is not known is the impact fatigue might have on the course of RA in the long term. In a review by Matcham and colleagues, the psychosocial factors associated with fatigue were considered in order to identify interventions for the symptom in RA (Matcham, Ali, Hotopf, & Chalder, 2015). They found a range of factors that could be grouped into six psychosocial categories: (1) mood, anxiety and depression, (2) cognitive deficits that are associated with RA, (3) cognitive deficits that are not associated with RA, (4) personality and common mental health disorders (RA-related cognitions, non-RA-related cognitions and personality characteristics), (5) stress and coping mechanisms and (6) social support and interpersonal relationships. As is seen in the case of CFS, low mood was associated with higher levels of fatigue and this relationship was found to be the most consistent across the different studies reviewed. Overall, their results suggested that interventions for fatigue in RA should focus on those which target anxiety, depression and mood together with the cognitive difficulties associated with RA (Matcham et al., 2015). In a cross-sectional study evaluating the relationship between work, mental health, physical health and fatigue in patients with RA, Żołnierczyk-Zreda et al. (2017) found that patients in employment reported lower levels of fatigue than those not in employment. They also found that this relationship was facilitated by better mental health but not by better physical health (Żołnierczyk-Zreda et al., 2017).

When we consider interventions for fatigue in RA, Cramp et al. (2013) reviewed 24 randomised control trials (RCT) where fatigue was included as an outcome measures. They identified two major types of intervention categories for RA namely, physical activity and psychosocial interventions (Cramp et al., 2013). The review concluded that physical activity and psychosocial interventions did help to reduce the fatigue experienced in RA but felt that the further research was required to determine the optimal non-pharmacological intervention.

Multiple Sclerosis

In order to address the fatigue experienced by patients with MS, researchers in New Zealand developed the Minimise Fatigue, Maximise Life: Creating Balance with Multiple Sclerosis (MFML) intervention (Mulligan, Wilkinson, & Snowdon, 2016). This is a group-based, fatigue self-management programme which is conducted over a six-week period. In their study, semi-structured interviews were conducted over the telephone with 23 patients who had completed the programme. In addition, they conducted a similar interview with 11 of these patients 3 months later. Mulligan and colleagues found that two themes emerged during the analysis of these outcome data: (1) the ability to affect behaviour in order to manage fatigue and (2) improvements in their day-to-day living. The benefits of the MFML program reported by patients included the successful development of fatigue self-management skills and their integration into their daily lives. This not only affected the individual, but also improved their ability to participate in family activities and engage more with the wider community (Mulligan et al., 2016). They also found that high levels of fatigue in MS were associated with high levels of depression and disability together with increased interference with usual activities, such as employment. Patients also reported that the fatigue experienced was unpredictable and intensified the other symptoms of MS, such as pain and lack of concentration.

When we consider interventions, Heine and colleagues reviewed 45 trials of exercise therapy (Heine, van de Port, Rietberg, van Wegen, & Kwakkel, 2015). The review concluded that although exercise therapy was helpful in reducing fatigue in MS and did not cause any exacerbation of the other symptoms of MS, the authors expressed concerns that there were some important methodological flaws to overcome. Further studies which addressed these concerns were recommended.

Parkinson's Disease

Apart from the motor symptoms associated with PD, fatigue is one of the most commonly reported problems. Again, the nature and mechanisms of the fatigue experienced is not completely understood. A study by Skorvanek and colleagues (2014) investigated the relationship between fatigue, apathy and depression in this illness together with other clinical and disease-related factors (Skorvanek et al., 2014). Their results suggested that patients with PD who were depressed were more likely to experience severe fatigue and apathy than those who were not depressed. In addition, fatigue, apathy and depression were distinct entities in PD.

When we consider interventions, Elbers and colleagues reviewed 11 intervention studies. Nine of the studies investigate the use of medication and two investigated the effect of exercise in reducing fatigue in PD (Elbers, Verhoef, van Wegen, Berendse, & Kwakkel, 2015). The authors could not make recommendations for any of the interventions reviewed and suggested that future research should focus on interventions to address behavioural or cognitive impairments in PD. They also highlighted the need for more appropriate self-related fatigue measures to be developed.

Cancer

Again, fatigue is a very common symptom in patients with cancer both during the course of the illness and during the treatment of the illness. It is also typically the most severe symptom reported by patients and the underlying mechanisms for the fatigue are unknown. In a study by Wang et al. (2014), the prevalence and nature of the fatigue experienced by patients was discussed. They found that patients were repeatedly reporting that fatigue was at such a level as to significantly impacting on their day-to-day living. Moderate/severe fatigue categories were statistically defined and reported by 45% of patients undergoing treatment. In patients with complete remission and those not receiving treatment, 29% also reported moderate/severe fatigue (Wang et al., 2014). In a study by Nishiura and colleagues (2015), the link between sleep disturbance and a range of psychological factors including fatigue in patients with lung cancer was investigated (Nishiura, Tamura, Nagai, & Matsushima, 2015). They found that of the 50 patients evaluated, 56% reported disturbed sleep. Patients with sleep disturbance reported higher levels of anxiety and depression, higher fatigue levels and higher levels of pain. There was also a link between impaired sleep and lower quality of life scores. Sedative hypnotic medication used to improve sleep did help patients fall asleep, but they did not improve sleep quality or decrease the daily functional impairment experienced by patients.

When we consider interventions, Goedendrop and colleagues (2009) reviewed 27 RCTs of psychosocial interventions for reducing fatigue experienced by adults during cancer treatment (Goedendrop, Gielissen, Verhagen, & Bleijenberg, 2009). The review concluded that seven of the studies reported significant effects of intervention on fatigue and only three provided evidence that the improvement was maintained over time. The authors reported limited evidence for the efficacy of psychosocial interventions for fatigue in adults during treatments for cancer and recommended further studies.

The findings of these reviews seem to follow a similar scenario as the one described previously in the medical history of CFS. That is to say that the fatigue experienced is of unknown origin but is thought to be as a result of several factors that collectively act to perpetuate it. In addition, methodological flaws are once again implicated in the failure to accurately identify the nature of fatigue experienced and there is a lack of coherent intervention strategies.

We can see from the reviews outlined above that, whilst persistent fatigue is acknowledged as a significant problem across a range of chronic conditions, it is not easy to measure or manage. With this in mind, we conducted an in-depth study of adults with DCD—a condition where fatigue as a secondary symptom is anecdotally reported—in order to investigate whether the CFS measures discussed in Chap. 2 could be used to measure fatigue in other conditions.

DEVELOPMENTAL COORDINATION DISORDER

DCD—sometimes referred to as dyspraxia—is one of the neurodevelopmental disorders and is characterised by severe impairments in motor proficiency which impact on normal day-to-day activities. The Diagnostic and Statistical Manual for Mental Disorders 5th edition (DSM 5) lists four diagnostic criteria for DCD. These include (1) motor performance that is substantially below expected levels, given the person's chronologic age and previous opportunities for skill acquisition, (2) that the motor impairment significantly and persistently interferes with activities of daily living or academic achievement, (3) onset of symptoms is in the early developmental period and (4) motor skill deficits are not better explained by intellectual disability or visual impairment and are not attributable to a neurological condition affecting movement (American Psychiatric Association, 2013). The prevalence of DCD in children is estimated to be between 1.4% and 19%, depending on the diagnostic criteria used (e.g. Lingam, Hunt, Golding, Jongmans, & Emond, 2009). Although not a precondition of DCD, children with the disorder experience high levels of fatigue. There have been a number of potential explanations for this, including less efficient patterns of motor movement during exercise (e.g. Silman, Cairney, Hay, Klentrou, & Faught, 2011). Such inefficiency likely results in higher energy expenditure which consequently accelerates the onset and development of fatigue. There have been several studies looking at the symptomology of DCD in children and, until relatively recently, the assumption has been that DCD was a condition only experienced during childhood. However, what was becoming increasingly clear was that this condition persists into adulthood. In addition, high levels of fatigue were increasingly being reported to clinicians as a significant impairment by adults with DCD. It was postulated that this fatigue could reflect the somatic manifestation of increased levels of anxiety and depression.

Based on the absence of research exploring the fatigue reported by adults with DCD, we used the subjective measures from the Cardiff CFS project (Smith et al., 1999; Thomas & Smith, 2006, 2009) to examine the nature of the fatigue associated with DCD. Adults with DCD were recruited via advertisement on the Dyspraxia Foundation's webpages and via email to international organisations and support groups. Typically developing (TD) controls were invited to participate in the research by the individuals with DCD participating in the study and staff at the host institution.

The subjective measures were administered to the DCD and TD groups via an online survey and included (1) the profile of fatigue-related symptoms (PFRS; Ray, Weir, Cullen, & Phillips, 1992), (2) state-trait anxiety inventory (STAI; Spielberger, Gorsuch, & Lushene, 1971), (3) Centre for Epidemiological Studies Depression Scale (CES-D; Radloff, 1977), (4) positive and negative affect (Zevon & Tellegen, 1982), (5) perceived stress scale (PSS; Cohen, Kamarck, & Mermelstein, 1983), (6) cognitive failures questionnaire (CFQ; Broadbent, Cooper, FitzGerald, & Parkes, 1982), (7) self-esteem (Fleming & Watts, 1980) and (8) symptoms checklist and sleep behaviour measure (Smith et al., 1999).

We can see from Table 4.1 that the adults with DCD reported higher levels of cognitive difficulties, fatigue, emotional distress and somatic

Table 4.1   Measures of fatigue and related symptoms for the DCD and TD adult groups

	DCD	TD	F(1, 88)
Cognitive difficulties	45.60	24.13	47.55; $p < 0.001$
Fatigue	49.11	28.47	29.24; $p < 0.001$
Emotional distress	60.04	37.16	22.39; $p < 0.001$
Somatic symptoms	44.78	30.38	14.34; $p < 0.001$
Anxiety	55.35	40.71	33.13; $p < 0.001$
Depression	48.62	35.81	22.39; $p < 0.001$
Positive affect	25.82	32.27	5.94; $p < 0.05$
Negative affect	29.80	16.22	22.63; $p < 0.001$
Perceived stress	34.09	24.29	21.45; $p < 0.001$
Cognitive failures (CFQ)	65.33	42.38	35.85; $p < 0.001$
Self-esteem	39.84	56.91	23.90; $p < 0.001$
Total symptoms	9.22	2.93	39.70; $p < 0.001$

symptoms than the TD group. They also reported higher levels of depression, anxiety, perceived stress, negative affect and overall symptoms than the TD group. In addition, the DCD group reported lower levels of (1) negative affect and (2) self-esteem.

When examining the individual items on the symptom checklist, not all 28 items were significantly different between the two groups. The DCD group reported higher levels of muscle pain, depression, anxiety, loss of concentration and loss of memory together with excessive fatigue (more than 50% of the time). In addition, physical weakness (more than 50% of the time), legs feeling 'heavy', bloated stomach, headache, acing heart and insomnia were also more likely to be reported in the DCD group. By ranking the items in order of prevalence, anxiety, sensitivity to noise, loss of concentration and muscle pain were the four most common symptoms reported by the DCD group.

We can see in Table 4.2 that the DCD group was significantly less likely to feel rested from sleep than the TD adults. However, there was no significant difference between the groups in terms of the number of hours slept per night (6–7 hours), difficulty falling asleep or problems with waking early.

Our findings clearly demonstrate the presence of marked fatigue in adults diagnosed with DCD. This finding gives credence to clinical observations that have been, up to now, anecdotal. The impact of the fatigue experienced is widespread, affecting a number of key indicators of well-being, such as mood, cognitive function, self-esteem and sleep. As this is the first study to examine fatigue in this group, such direct comparisons cannot be made. However, given the model used in this study, it is possible to explore similarities between the DCD groups here and our previously published data on CFS groups—discussed in Chap. 2.

Table 4.2 Measure of sleep behaviour ('how often do you feel rested from sleep')

	DCD (%)	TD (%)	Sig.
Rested from sleep			
Never	5.7	5.8	$\chi^2 = 10.29$; $df = 1$; $p < 0.05$
Almost never	28.3	17.3	
Sometimes	45.3	26.9	
Fairly often	17.0	38.5	
Very often	3.8	11.5	

Table 4.3 Measures of fatigue and related symptoms for the DCD and CFS groups

	DCD	CFS
Cognitive difficulties	45.20	51.48
Fatigue	49.32	70.36
Emotional distress	59.43	57.96
Somatic symptoms	44.27	64.37
Anxiety	55.20	54.49
Depression	48.52	48.73
Positive affect	25.95	23.99
Negative affect	29.39	28.75
Perceived stress	33.95	32.55
Cognitive failures	64.98	59.37
Self-esteem	40.04	45.81
Total symptoms	9.23	16.49

We, therefore, also recruited a group of individuals with CFS. When we compare the DCD and CFS groups we find that there are differences and similarities.

We can see in Table 4.3 that, in terms of differences, the DCD group report significantly lower levels of cognitive difficulties, fatigue, somatic symptoms and total symptoms than the CFS group. However, they did report similar levels of anxiety, depression, perceived stress, emotional distress, cognitive failures, negative and positive affects and self-esteem (Thomas & Christopher, 2017).

The importance of our findings is that we have been able to employ the subjective measures used previously in our CFS research (Thomas & Smith, 2008) to investigate fatigue in another patient group who were increasingly reporting its impact on their day-to-day lives. We propose that the behavioural therapies discussed in Chap. 3 could be more generally used across a range of conditions with fatigue as a co-occurring symptom, but it would be of interest to see if this is currently happening in practice.

SUMMARY

We can see from the studies outlined in this chapter that fatigue presents as a significant symptom in a range of chronic conditions, it is of unknown aetiology but causes substantial problems in day-to-day living. Problems including depression and poor sleep quality were also associated with fatigue in these conditions. The systematic reviews indicate that although there have been many efficacy studies focussing on interventions for fatigue in individual conditions, there is a need for the development of more generalisable programmes for its management. Each of the review authors also highlight the heterogeneity of the individual conditions and methodological flaws as important factors to be considered in future research.

In previous research, we developed a range of subjective and objective measures which we used to quantify the symptoms associated with CFS and that were sensitive enough to evaluate the efficacy of interventions for the illness. We have now used the subjective measures to quantify fatigue in another disorder, DCD. Our study provided evidence of the high levels of fatigue, somatic symptoms, emotional distress and cognitive difficulties experienced by adults with this disorder. The checklist provides evidence of the myriad symptoms experienced by those with DCD and further highlights their similarity to the CFS group. Higher levels of perceived stress and negative affect together with low positive affect were also reported. Sleep plays a vital role in resolving fatigue and as such is a major factor for consideration when diagnosing such conditions. Findings from the current study suggest that, although those with DCD are sleeping for the same number of hours per night as the TD group and are not having problems falling asleep or waking early, they are in fact not feeling rested by sleep. Such subjective reporting is likely to contribute to the fatigue experienced by this group.

Our efficacy studies for interventions in CFS that were discussed in Chap. 3 together with findings from the DCD study have implications for future research into the evaluation of interventions for fatigue across a range of chronic conditions.

References

American Psychiatric Association. (2013). *Diagnostic and statistical manual for mental disorders, 5th edition (DSM-5)*. Arlington, VA: American Psychiatric Publishing.

Arthritis Research UK. Retrieved March 2018, from www.arthritisresearchuk.org.

Broadbent, D. E., Cooper, P. F., FitzGerald, P., & Parkes, K. R. (1982). The cognitive failures questionnaire (CFQ) and its correlates. *The British Journal of Clinical Psychology/The British Psychological Society, 21*(Pt. 1), 1–16.

Cella, D., Lai, J.-S., Jensen, S., Christodoulou, C., Junghaenel, D., Reeve, B., et al. (2016). Clinical validity of the PROMIS® fatigue item bank across diverse clinical samples. *Journal of Clinical Epidemiology, 73*, 128–134.

Cohen, S., Kamarck, T., & Mermelstein, R. (1983). A global measure of perceived stress. *Journal of Health and Social Behavior, 24*(4), 385–396.

Cramp, F., Hewlett, S., Almeida, C., Kirwan, J., Choy, E., Chalder, T., et al. (2013). Non-pharmacological interventions for fatigue in rheumatoid arthritis. *Cochrane Database of Systematic Reviews.*

Elbers, R., Verhoef, J., van Wegen, E., Berendse, H., & Kwakkel, G. (2015). Interventions for fatigue in Parkinson's disease. *Cochrane Database of Systematic Reviews.*

Fleming, J. S., & Watts, W. A. (1980). The dimensionality of self-esteem: Some results of a college sample. *Journal of Personality and Social Psychology, 39*(5), 921–929.

Goedendrop, M., Gielissen, M., Verhagen, C., & Bleijenberg, G. (2009). Psychosocial interventions for reducing fatigue during cancer treatment in adults. *Cochrane Database of Systematic Reviews.*

Heine, M., van de Port, I., Rietberg, M., van Wegen, E., & Kwakkel, G. (2015). Exercise therapy for fatigue in multiple sclerosis. *Cochrane Database of Systematic Reviews.*

Lingam, R., Hunt, L., Golding, J., Jongmans, M., & Emond, A. (2009). Prevalence of developmental coordination disorder using the DSM-IV at 7 years of age: A UK population–based study. *Pediatrics, 123*(4), e693–e700.

Matcham, F., Ali, S., Hotopf, M., & Chalder, T. (2015). Psychological correlates of fatigue in rheumatoid arthritis: A systematic review. *Clinical Psychology Review, 39*, 16–29.

Mulligan, H., Wilkinson, A., & Snowdon, J. (2016). Perceived impact of a self-management program for fatigue in multiple sclerosis a qualitative study. *International Journal of Multiple Sclerosis, 18*, 27–32.

Nicholson, K., Stewart, M., & Thind, A. (2015). Examining the symptom of fatigue in primary care: A comparative study using electronic medical records. *Journal of Innovative Health Information, 22*, 235–243.

Nishiura, M., Tamura, A., Nagai, H., & Matsushima, E. (2015). Assessment of sleep disturbance in lung cancer patients: Relationship between sleep disturbance and pain, fatigue, quality of life, and psychological distress. *Palliative and Supportive Care, 13*, 575–581.

Silman, A., Cairney, J., Hay, J., Klentrou, P., & Faught, B. E. (2011). Role of physical activity and perceived adequacy on peak aerobic power in children with developmental coordination disorder. *Human Movement Science, 30*(3), 672–681. https://doi.org/10.1016/j.humov.2010.08.005

Skorvanek, M., Gdovinova, Z., Rosenberger, J., Ghorbani Saeedian, R., Nagyova, I., Groothoff, J., et al. (2014). The associations between fatigue, apathy, and depression in Parkinson's disease. *Acta Neurologica Scandinavica, 13*, 80–87.

Smith, A., Borysiewicz, L., Pollock, J., Thomas, M., Perry, K., & Llewelyn, M. (1999). Acute fatigue in chronic fatigue syndrome patients. *Psychological Medicine, 29,* 283.

Spielberger, C., Gorsuch, R., & Lushene, R. (1971). *STAI manual for the state-trait anxiety inventory.* Palo Alto, CA: Consulting Psychologists Press.

Radloff, L. S. (1977). The CES-D scale: A self-report depression scale for research in the general population. *Applied Psychological Measurement, 1*(3), 385–401. https://doi.org/10.1177/014662167700100306

Ray, C., Weir, W. R. C., Cullen, S., & Phillips, S. (1992). Illness perception and symptom components in chronic fatigue syndrome. *Journal of Psychosomatic Research, 36*(3), 243–256.

Thomas, M., & Christopher, G. (2017). Fatigue in developmental coordination disorder: An exploratory study in adults. *Fatigue: Biomedicine, Health & Behavior.* https://doi.org/10.1080/21641846.2018.1419564

Thomas, M., & Smith, A. (2006). An investigation of the long-term benefits of antidepressant medication in the recovery of patients with chronic fatigue syndrome. *Human Psychopharmacology: Clinical and Experimental, 21*(8), 503–509. https://doi.org/10.1002/hup.805

Thomas, M., & Smith, A. (2008). An investigation into the cognitive deficits associated with chronic fatigue syndrome. *The Open Neurology Journal, 3,* 13–23. https://doi.org/10.2174/1874205X00903010013

Wang, X., Fengmin, Z., Fisch, M., O'Mara, A., Cella, D., Mendoza, T., et al. (2014). Prevalence and characteristics of moderate to severe fatigue: A multicentre study in cancer patients and survivors. *Cancer, 120,* 425–432.

Zevon, M. A., & Tellegen, A. (1982). The structure of mood change: An idiographic/nomothetic analysis. *Journal of Personality and Social Psychology, 43*(1), 111–122.

Żołnierczyk-Zreda, D., Jędryka-Góral, A., Bugajska, J., Bedyńska, S., Brzosko, M., & Pazdur, J. (2017). The relationship between work, mental health, physical health, and fatigue in patients with rheumatoid arthritis: A cross-sectional study. *Journal of Health Psychology.* https://doi.org/10.1177/1359105317727842

CHAPTER 5

Fatigue: An Overview of Chronic Fatigue and Recommendations for Future Research

Abstract This chapter provides any overview of fatigue including a medical history of CFS, an investigation into the symptoms and cognitive impairments associated with it and a range of interventions—both pharmacological and behavioural—that have been shown to manage the condition. The chapter also provides an overview of a range of chronic conditions where fatigue is reported by patients as a significant but secondary symptom of unknown aetiology. This includes rheumatoid arthritis, multiple sclerosis, Parkinson's disease and cancer. Interventions for these conditions are also discussed. A study investigating the fatigue in adults with developmental coordination disorder is also discussed. The chapter ends with recommendations for future research regarding fatigue—including fatigue in older adults.

Keywords Chronic fatigue syndrome • Fatigue • Chronic conditions • Intervention • Symptoms • Older adults

OVERVIEW OF CHRONIC FATIGUE

According to Landmark-Høyvik and colleagues, 'fatigue can be conceptualised as a final common end point for psychological and biological processes. Fatigue is therefore both heterogeneous (occurring across different conditions) and multifactorial' (Landmark-Høyvik et al., 2009).

© The Author(s) 2018
M. Thomas, *"Tired all the Time"*,
https://doi.org/10.1007/978-3-319-93913-1_5

In order to bring the topics covered previously in this Pivot into context, this section will provide a brief overview of Chaps. 1, 2, 3 and 4.

Summary of Chapter 1: A Medical History of Chronic Fatigue

This chapter looked at the medical history of chronic fatigue from neurasthenia in the 1800s to chronic fatigue syndrome (CFS) in the present day (Wessely, 1991; Thomas, 2009) together with three pivotal reports that aimed at bringing consensus to both medical professionals and researchers in the field. The reports made recommendations about the ways in which the research should develop, such as the need to identify and investigate factors responsible for both causing and perpetuating the illness (Sharpe et al., 1991) and urged clinicians to accept the existence of the illness, provide a service for patients and take steps to manage patients in their care (Royal Colleges of Physicians, Psychiatrists and General Practitioners, 1996). Recommendations were made that cognitive behaviour therapy (CBT) and graded exercise were the most successful methods for managing symptoms of the illness (CFS/ME Working Group, 2002).

Summary of Chapter 2: Chronic Fatigue Syndrome

This chapter looked at how we addressed the recommendations made in the 1991 Guidelines for Research (Sharpe et al., 1991). We conducted a three-year longitudinal study that looked at the prognosis of CFS and the symptoms associated with it along with factors which might perpetuate the condition. Full recovery from the untreated illness was uncommon (Thomas & Smith, 2006) and individuals with CFS reported numerous physical and mental symptoms and problems with sleep quality. We also identified the presence of co-morbid mood disorder in this patient group together with lower levels of alertness, less enjoyment from life and higher levels of anxiety. One of the most important findings was the identification of the cognitive deficits using objective measures of cognition (Thomas & Smith, 2008).

Summary of Chapter 3: Healthcare Provision for CFS

This chapter looked at underlying beliefs about the condition in both patients and GPs (Thomas & Smith, 2005) in light of the report by the Royal Colleges (Royal Colleges of Physicians, Psychiatrists and General

Practitioners, 1996). We then went on to look at symptom management for CFS. We found that antidepressant medication, especially selective sero-tonin re-uptake inhibitors (SSRIs), did benefit patients (Thomas & Smith, 2006). In response to the CFS/ME Working Group report (2002), we also conducted two efficacy studies. They first evaluated an multi-convergent therapy (MCT), which included CBT and graded exercise (Thomas, Sadlier, & Smith 2006, 2008), and the second looked at the counselling services and rehabilitation courses provided by Action for ME (AfME) (Thomas & Smith, 2007). Our findings indicated that MCT resulted in improvements in cognitive performance and reductions in illness severity, and that these improvements were maintained six months after the therapy and also three years later (Smith, Thomas, & Sadlier, 2009). We also found that AfME's services were of benefit to patients with CFS in areas such as lowering levels of fatigue and physical symptoms (Thomas & Smith, 2007).

Summary of Chapter 4: Persistent Fatigue in Chronic Conditions

This chapter looked at the prevalence of persistent fatigue in chronic con-ditions. Two large-scale studies in Canada (Nicholson, Stewart, & Thind, 2015) and the USA (Cella et al., 2016) highlighted the prevalence and impact of fatigue in their primary care systems. The symptoms associated with the fatigue experienced by patients with rheumatoid arthritis (RA), multiple sclerosis (MS), Parkinson's disease (PD) and cancer were explored together with efficacy studies to manage the fatigue in each condition. The four reviews all concluded that the outcome measures currently being used were not sensitive to fatigue and that current management strategies were not very successful. Using the measures discussed in Chap. 2 we were able to quantify fatigue in DCD where fatigue is not the primary presenting symptom (Thomas & Christopher, 2017). Our findings have implications for possible future efficacy intervention studies for the management of fatigue across a range of chronic conditions.

FUTURE RESEARCH

Preliminary work aiming to identify possible subgroups in CFS led us to investigate alexithymia and emotional intelligence, both of which are known to highlight specific therapeutic needs for patient groups. For example, a difficulty specifying particular emotions—a deficit central to alexithymia—has been shown to be linked to increased use of medical care

(Lumley & Norman, 1996). When splitting the CFS patients into those who score either high or low on alexithymia, we found distinct differences between the groups concerning how well they are able to deal with the types of challenges we all face in our everyday lives. Those in the high alexithymia group are more likely to view problems as a threat and tend to respond to these situations impulsively or avoid responding at all. This mindset is associated with negative outcomes to social problem situations and a tendency to either give up or enlist the help of others. This was linked to our finding that individuals with high alexithymia scores tend to experience distress when witnessing someone else's upset. If an individual lacks the ability to use compensatory strategies, it is more likely that they will give up following a failed attempt to solve a problem. We found that emotional intelligence positively correlates with effective social problem solving. In addition, when looking at the high and low alexithymia groups, emotional intelligence scores were significantly lower in the high alexithymia group. This suggests that individual with low emotional intelligence scores are more likely to coincide with maladaptive problem-solving orientation and styles (Christopher & Thomas, 2009). Our sample size for this study was low and future research would include further data collection in order to fully explore the impact of alexithymia on social problem solving in CFS. The objective being to provide valuable insight into the mechanisms underpinning CFS, with the potential to inform future interventions to help address the heterogeneous symptomatology seen in this group. The outcomes are likely to be of greatest importance for the early stages of the condition in terms of the selection of the most appropriate form of intervention. In addition, we may be able to describe a subgrouping of CFS based on alexithymia/emotional intelligence and to identify, through the use of regression analyses, variables which can be seen to predict significantly membership to these subgroups, thereby offering the potential to offer more personalised interventions depending on the individual needs of the patient.

Persistent fatigue is an increasingly reported problem in primary care, being linked to other chronic conditions such as RA, MS, PD and cancer. For each of these conditions, fatigue is a significant problem for patients. However, in all such cases its aetiology is unknown and is distinct from the diagnostic criteria of these illnesses. In studies of RA, it has been suggested that anxiety, depression, mood and cognitive impairments as areas to be considered in the management of the fatigue experienced by people with this condition (Matcham, Ali, Hotopf, & Chalder, 2015). In MS, fatigue has been linked to levels of disability and depression together with problems in day-to-day functioning, including employment (Mulligan, Wilkinson, & Snowdon, 2016). Research into the PD suggested that heightened levels of fatigue were associated with increased depression (Skorvanek et al., 2014). The fatigue experienced by patients with cancer was linked to sleep disturbance (Nishiura, Tamura, Nagai, & Matsushima, 2015).

We can see that the factors associated with the persistent fatigue experienced in the chronic conditions outlined above reflect the findings from our CFS studies. However, when we consider the findings from the systematic reviews discussed in Chap. 4, there is currently no generalisable intervention to alleviate fatigue across a range of conditions. In addition, recommendations were made for the use of more rigorous outcome measures to evaluate possible interventions by the authors of the each of the reviews (Cramp et al., 2013; Heine, van de Port, Rietberg, van Wegen, & Kwakkel, 2015; Elbers, Verhoef, van Wegen, Berendse, & Kwakkel, 2015; Goedendrop, Gielissen, Verhagen, & Bleijenberg, 2009).

Future research will focus on using the objective and subjective measures developed for the CFS project to develop and evaluate interventions for fatigue associated with a range of conditions in the primary care setting. One-to-one interventions such as MCT are costly to administer in an already strained health service and are time consuming for both therapist and patient. In order to reduce the costs of fatigue interventions, it would be important to develop and trial online versions of the therapy sessions. This has already proved successful in the case of CBT. We would then trial the online version using the measures developed previously (Thomas & Smith, 2008). To make this process more accessible to those taking part in the research, we would also administer the evaluation measures online.

Fatigue is also one of the most frequent symptoms reported by older adults and could result in a loss of independence together with decreased physical activity and functional decline. In many cases clinicians will find an underlying physical or psychiatric cause and offer appropriate treatment. However, increasingly older people report complaints of fatigue with no known aetiology and this should not be solely attributed to 'just getting old'. We are all aware that people are living longer, and it will be important to investigate how we can best manage fatigue in older adults in primary care. We have seen how fatigue can impact on aspects of daily living and addressing its management will be vital to maintain the quality of life and independence of an increasingly ageing population.

In addition, it may be necessary to offer strategies to manage acute fatigue. Acute fatigue is very much seen as a protective symptom which alerts us that we need to rest. Acute fatigue is usually characterised by rapid onset and short duration and is a normal response to over-exertion. However, episodes of acute fatigue can occur without a precipitating cause. This is another topic of interest for future research. In other words, to investigate the possibility of developing a way of intervening when episodes of acute fatigue occur in older adults.

As discussed throughout this Pivot, there remains inconsistency in the research literature on both the identification of and interventions for fatigue. We continue to work towards solving the problems that persistent fatigue presents across a range of conditions.

REFERENCES

Cella, D., Lai, J.-S., Jensen, S., Christodoulou, C., Junghaenel, D., Reeve, B., et al. (2016). Clinical validity of the PROMIS® fatigue item bank across diverse clinical samples. *Journal of Clinical Epidemiology, 73*, 128–134.

CFS/ME Working Group. (2002). *Report to the Chief Medical Officer of an independent working group*. London: Department of Health.

Christopher, G., & Thomas, M. (2009). Social problem solving and Chronic Fatigue Syndrome. *Stress & Health, 25*, 161–169.

Cramp, F., Hewlett, S., Almeida, C., Kirwan, J., Choy, E., Chalder, T., et al. (2013). Non-pharmacological interventions for fatigue in rheumatoid arthritis. *Cochrane Database of Systematic Reviews*.

Elbers, R., Verhoef, J., van Wegen, E., Berendse, H., & Kwakkel, G. (2015). Interventions for fatigue in Parkinson's disease. *Cochrane Database of Systematic Reviews*.

Goedendrop, M., Gielissen, M., Verhagen, C., & Bleijenberg, G. (2009). Psychosocial interventions for reducing fatigue during cancer treatment in adults. *Cochrane Database of Systematic Reviews*.

Heine, M., van de Port, I., Rietberg, M., van Wegen, E., & Kwakkel, G. (2015). Exercise therapy for fatigue in multiple sclerosis. *Cochrane Database of Systematic Reviews*.

Landmark-Høyvik, H., Reinertsen, K., Loge, J., Fosså, S., Børresen-Dale, A., & Dumeaux, V. (2009). Alterations of gene expression in blood cells associated with chronic fatigue in breast cancer survivors. *Journal of Pharmacogenomics, 9*, 333–340.

Lumley, M., & Norman, S. (1996). Alexithymia and health care utilization. *Psychosomatic Medicine, 58*, 197–202.

Matcham, F., Ali, S., Hotopf, M., & Chalder, T. (2015). Psychological correlates of fatigue in rheumatoid arthritis: A systematic review. *Clinical Psychology Review, 39*, 16–29.

Mulligan, H., Wilkinson, A., & Snowdon, J. (2016). Perceived impact of a self-management program for fatigue in multiple sclerosis a qualitative study. *International Journal of Multiple Sclerosis, 18*, 27–32.

Nicholson, K., Stewart, M., & Thind, A. (2015). Examining the symptom of fatigue in primary care: A comparative study using electronic medical records. *Journal of Innovative Health Information, 22*, 235–243.

Nishiura, M., Tamura, A., Nagai, H., & Matsushima, E. (2015). Assessment of sleep disturbance in lung cancer patients: Relationship between sleep disturbance and pain, fatigue, quality of life, and psychological distress. *Palliative and Supportive Care, 13*, 575–581.

Report of the Royal Colleges of Physicians, Psychiatrists and General Practitioners. (1996). *Chronic Fatigue Syndrome*. London: RCP.

Sharpe, M. C., Archard, L. C., Banatvala, J. E., Borysiewicz, L. K., Clare, A. W., David, A., et al. (1991). A report—Chronic fatigue syndrome: Guidelines for research. *Journal of the Royal Society of Medicine, 84*, 118–121.

Skorvanek, M., Gdovinova, Z., Rosenberger, J., Ghorbani Saeedian, R., Nagyova, I., Groothoff, J., et al. (2014). The associations between fatigue, apathy, and depression in Parkinson's disease. *Acta Neurologica Scandinavica, 13*, 80–87.

Smith, A., Thomas, M., & Sadlier, M. (2009). Multi-convergent therapy: A possible intervention to aid return to work. *Occupational Health at Work, 6*, 30–32.

Thomas, M. (2009). *Exploring the beliefs and underlying functional deficits associated with CFS and the identification of predictors of recovery and successful illness management*. PhD thesis, University of Wales.

Thomas, M., & Christopher, G. (2017). Fatigue in developmental coordination disorder: An exploratory study in adults. *Fatigue: Biomedicine, Health & Behavior*. https://doi.org/10.1080/21641846.2018.1419564

Thomas, M., Sadlier, M., & Smith, A. (2006). The effect of Multi Convergent Therapy on the psychopathology, mood and performance of Chronic Fatigue Syndrome patients: A preliminary study. *Counselling and Psychotherapy Research, 6*, 91–99.

Thomas, M., Sadlier, M., & Smith, A. (2008). A multi-convergent approach to the rehabilitation of patients with Chronic Fatigue Syndrome: A comparative study. *Physiotherapy, 94*, 35–42.

Thomas, M., & Smith, A. (2005). Primary healthcare provision and Chronic Fatigue Syndrome: A survey of patients' and general practitioners' beliefs. *BMC Family Practice, 6*, 49. https://doi.org/10.1186/1471-2296-6-49

Thomas, M., & Smith, A. (2006). An investigation of the long-term benefits of antidepressant medication in the recovery of patients with chronic fatigue syndrome. *Human Psychopharmacology: Clinical and Experimental, 21*(8), 503–509. https://doi.org/10.1002/hup.805

Thomas, M. A., & Smith, A. P. (2007). The evaluation of counselling and rehabilitation courses for Chronic Fatigue Syndrome patients. *Counselling and Psychotherapy Research, 7*, 164–171.

Thomas, M., & Smith, A. (2008). An investigation into the cognitive deficits associated with Chronic Fatigue Syndrome. *Open Neurology Journal, 2*, 78–88.

Wessely, S. (1991). History of postviral fatigue syndrome. *British Medical Bulletin, 47*, 919–941.